Methylene Blue Healing Bible

Uncover the Limitless Power of This Groundbreaking Molecule to Naturally Revitalize Your Body, Strengthen Immunity, and Pave the Way to Lifelong Vitality and Well-Being

Elvira Lawson

Methylene Blue Healing Bible

Printed in the United States of America

TABLE OF CONTENT

CHAPTER 1: INTRODUCTION TO METHYLENE BLUE

What if a single compound, discovered over a century ago, held the potential to transform your energy levels, sharpen your mind, and unlock new realms of vitality? Welcome to the world of methylene blue—a substance that began its journey as a humble textile dye and has evolved into one of the most fascinating tools in modern health and biohacking.

THE HISTORY AND EVOLUTION OF METHYLENE BLUE

To understand why methylene blue is gaining attention as a groundbreaking tool for health and biohacking, it helps to explore its fascinating history—a journey that spans over a century, moving from textile factories to cutting-edge medical research.

The Discovery of Methylene Blue

The story of methylene blue begins in 1876 when a German chemist named Heinrich Caro synthesized it as part of efforts to create vibrant, affordable dyes for the booming textile industry. Its striking blue hue quickly made it popular for coloring fabrics, but scientists soon noticed something intriguing: methylene blue's chemical properties went far beyond its role as a dye. During this time, the scientific community was beginning to explore how certain compounds interacted with living organisms. Methylene blue stood out because of its ability to bind to biological molecules and its remarkable visibility under a microscope, making it an ideal tool for studying cells.

A Medical Breakthrough

In the late 19th century, researchers began to test methylene blue in medical applications. Paul Ehrlich, a German physician and scientist, recognized its potential for staining cells and bacteria, allowing doctors to identify disease-causing organisms more easily. This innovation marked methylene blue's entry into the medical field.

Ehrlich's experiments went further. In 1891, he discovered that methylene blue could kill the parasite responsible for malaria. This was a groundbreaking moment in medicine—it was the first synthetic drug ever used to treat an infectious disease. Although eventually replaced by more effective treatments, methylene blue's success against malaria laid the foundation for modern pharmacology, earning it a place in medical history.

From Diagnostic Tool to Cellular Support

Throughout the 20th century, methylene blue's applications continued to expand. It became a staple in diagnostic medicine, used to stain tissues during surgery and to detect certain diseases. Meanwhile, scientists explored its effects on human cells, particularly its interactions with mitochondria—the tiny "power plants" in our cells responsible for producing energy.

Mitochondria produce energy in the form of ATP (adenosine triphosphate) through a process called cellular respiration. This process relies on the flow of electrons, which can sometimes go awry, causing oxidative stress and damage. Methylene blue has a unique ability to act as an electron carrier, stabilizing the energy production process and reducing oxidative stress. This discovery opened the door to methylene blue's potential as a therapeutic agent for conditions related to mitochondrial dysfunction, including fatigue, neurodegenerative diseases, and aging.

A New Wave of Interest

In recent decades, methylene blue has experienced a resurgence, thanks to growing interest in biohacking and wellness optimization. Researchers have demonstrated its benefits as a neuroprotective agent, capable of enhancing cognitive function and protecting against conditions like Alzheimer's and Parkinson's diseases. It has also been shown to improve energy levels, combat oxidative stress, and even reverse some of the visible and invisible effects of aging. Biohackers and longevity enthusiasts have embraced methylene blue as a tool for optimizing both physical and mental performance. Its ability to boost mitochondrial function, reduce fatigue, and enhance focus has made it a popular choice among those looking to unlock their full potential.

From the Past to the Future

The evolution of methylene blue—from a textile dye to a pioneering medical treatment and now a cutting-edge wellness tool—is a testament to its versatility and untapped potential. Its journey reflects the intersection of science, innovation, and the timeless human pursuit of better health and performance. As you explore its applications throughout this book, you'll discover how methylene blue can play a transformative role in your own journey toward vitality, longevity, and resilience.

WHY METHYLENE BLUE IS A GAME-CHANGER IN HEALTH AND WELLNESS

In a world filled with supplements, therapies, and biohacking tools promising improved health and longevity, few stand out as genuinely transformative. Methylene blue is one of them. Its unique mechanisms, broad benefits, and potential to address root causes of many health challenges make it a true game-changer.

Here's why.

1. **A Cellular Energy Booster:** At the core of every cell in your body are mitochondria, often referred to as the "power plants" of cells. These tiny structures are responsible for producing energy in the form of ATP (adenosine triphosphate). However, as we age, or due to stress, poor lifestyle choices, and chronic conditions, mitochondria can become less efficient, leading to energy deficits. Methylene blue works at the mitochondrial level to optimize energy production. It acts as an electron carrier in the electron transport chain, a key process in cellular respiration. Think of it as an energy "backup generator" that steps in to smooth out inefficiencies, helping your cells produce more energy while reducing the byproducts of oxidative stress. This unique ability makes methylene blue a powerful tool for overcoming chronic fatigue and restoring vitality.

2. **Cognitive Enhancer and Brain Protector:** Your brain, with its high demand for energy, benefits immensely from methylene blue's mitochondrial support. But its effects on cognition go further. Methylene blue improves blood flow and oxygen delivery to the brain, which enhances focus, memory, and mental clarity. Moreover, it acts as a neuroprotective agent. By neutralizing free radicals and reducing oxidative damage, methylene blue protects neurons from the wear and tear of aging, stress, and inflammation. Research has also shown its potential to slow the progression of neurodegenerative diseases like Alzheimer's and Parkinson's by supporting cellular repair mechanisms and reducing the buildup of harmful proteins in the brain. For anyone dealing with brain fog, memory lapses, or cognitive decline, methylene blue offers a beacon of hope.

3. **Anti-Aging at the Cellular Level:** Aging is inevitable, but the speed and way it affects your body are not. A significant part of aging involves damage caused by oxidative stress—an imbalance between free radicals and the body's ability to neutralize them. Methylene blue, with its potent antioxidant properties, helps restore this balance. It works by scavenging harmful reactive oxygen species (ROS) and supporting the repair of damaged cells. Additionally, methylene blue can increase the lifespan of mitochondria and improve their function, which is critical for slowing cellular aging. The result? Healthier cells, more youthful skin, and a body that feels and performs better over time.

4. **Immune and Overall Health Support:** Methylene blue's benefits don't stop at energy and cognition. It has been shown to bolster immune resilience by reducing inflammation and aiding in the repair of cellular damage caused by illness or stress. Its ability to improve blood oxygenation and circulation also supports cardiovascular health and physical endurance. For individuals dealing with chronic conditions like autoimmune disorders or neurodegenerative diseases, methylene blue offers a non-invasive, science-backed way to promote healing and recovery.

5. **A Tool for Modern Wellness:** Methylene blue isn't just a treatment—it's a proactive tool for thriving in today's fast-paced world. Whether you're a busy professional seeking sustained focus, a biohacker looking to optimize performance, or someone trying to overcome fatigue and feel their best, methylene blue addresses foundational health challenges that other supplements often miss.

Why It Matters to You

Unlike many health trends that offer surface-level solutions, methylene blue targets the root causes of energy depletion, cognitive decline, and aging. Its ability to enhance cellular efficiency, protect the brain, and reduce oxidative stress makes it one of the most versatile and impactful tools available today. By integrating methylene blue into your wellness journey, you're not just adding another supplement—you're empowering your body and mind to function at their peak. The benefits are profound: more energy, sharper thinking, healthier aging, and an overall sense of vitality. Methylene blue is not just a game-changer; it's a life-changer.

CHAPTER 2: THE SCIENCE BEHIND METHYLENE BLUE

In this foundational chapter, we'll explore the powerful science behind methylene blue and its transformative effects on the body. First, we'll unravel the mysteries of mitochondria, your cells' energy factories, and why their health is crucial for vitality and longevity. Next, we'll dive into methylene blue's unique mechanisms of action, from boosting mitochondrial efficiency to acting as an electron donor. Finally, we'll examine its potent antioxidant properties, explaining how it combats oxidative stress and supports cellular repair. By the end of this chapter, you'll understand why methylene blue is a cutting-edge tool for optimizing energy, cognition, and overall wellness.

UNDERSTANDING CELLULAR ENERGY AND MITOCHONDRIAL FUNCTION

To understand why methylene blue is such a powerful tool for health, it's essential to first grasp how your body produces energy. At the heart of this process are tiny organelles within your cells called mitochondria—often referred to as the "powerhouses" of the cell. These small but mighty structures are responsible for generating energy in a form that your body can use: a molecule called adenosine triphosphate (ATP).

Step 1: The Role of Mitochondria in Energy Production

Think of mitochondria as power plants, converting raw materials (the food you eat and the oxygen you breathe) into usable energy. This conversion happens through a process called cellular respiration, which takes place in several steps:

1. **Breaking Down Food Molecules:** When you eat, carbohydrates, fats, and proteins are broken down into smaller molecules such as glucose or fatty acids. These molecules enter your cells and are processed further by the mitochondria.

2. **The Electron Transport Chain:** Inside the mitochondria, the real magic happens. Electrons from these molecules are passed through a series of proteins called the electron transport chain (ETC). This chain works like a conveyor belt, moving electrons from one protein to another. As this happens, a flow of protons generates a kind of "energy gradient," similar to water building up behind a dam.

3. **Generating ATP:** At the end of this chain, an enzyme called ATP synthase uses the energy from the gradient to convert a molecule called ADP into ATP—the energy currency your cells need to function.

This process is remarkably efficient, producing the energy that powers everything from muscle contractions to brain activity and even the repair of damaged tissues.

Step 2: Why Mitochondrial Health Matters

When mitochondria are healthy and functioning properly, your body feels energized, your brain stays sharp, and your cells repair themselves efficiently. However, mitochondria are also highly sensitive to damage from stress, aging, toxins, and poor lifestyle choices. Here's what happens when they aren't working optimally:

1. **Energy Deficit:** When mitochondria are damaged, they can't produce ATP as effectively. This can leave you feeling tired, mentally foggy, and unable to recover from physical or emotional stress.

2. **Oxidative Stress:** The electron transport chain occasionally leaks unstable molecules called free radicals, which can damage cells if not neutralized. Over time, this oxidative stress can harm your mitochondria and other cellular components, accelerating aging and contributing to chronic diseases.

3. **Mitochondrial Dysfunction:** When mitochondria are overwhelmed by damage, they become less efficient and may even die. This dysfunction is linked to many health problems, including fatigue, brain fog, neurodegenerative diseases, and cardiovascular issues.

Step 3: How Mitochondria Impact Your Everyday Life

Mitochondria aren't just abstract cellular components—they directly affect how you feel and perform every day. For example:

- **Energy Levels:** Whether you wake up refreshed or struggle through the day depends largely on mitochondrial efficiency.
- **Cognitive Function:** Your brain requires massive amounts of energy to think, focus, and process information. Healthy mitochondria are key to mental clarity and memory.
- **Aging and Recovery:** The aging process is deeply tied to mitochondrial function. Maintaining strong mitochondria can slow the visible and invisible effects of aging, while aiding faster recovery from exercise or illness.

Step 4: Methylene Blue's Role in Supporting Mitochondria

Mitochondria are the energy powerhouses of your cells, converting nutrients and oxygen into ATP, the energy currency your body relies on. When mitochondria are functioning well, you feel energized, mentally sharp, and physically strong. However, stress, aging, toxins, and illness can disrupt this process, leading to mitochondrial dysfunction—a root cause of fatigue, brain fog, and chronic health issues. This is where methylene blue shines as a mitochondrial enhancer.

First, methylene blue acts as an electron donor, ensuring the smooth flow of electrons along the mitochondrial electron transport chain. Think of it as a helper that bridges gaps in the chain, enabling your cells to produce energy more efficiently. Second, it optimizes oxygen utilization. When oxygen levels are low or mitochondria struggle to use it effectively, methylene blue steps in to support energy production even under less-than-ideal conditions.

Finally, methylene blue combats oxidative stress—damage caused by free radicals generated during energy production. By neutralizing these harmful molecules, it protects your mitochondria and supports cellular repair. By enhancing mitochondrial function, methylene blue doesn't just increase energy—it boosts resilience, sharpens mental clarity, and promotes overall vitality, making it a cornerstone of health optimization.

HOW METHYLENE BLUE WORKS: MECHANISMS OF ACTION

Methylene blue is a compound with remarkable properties that make it a powerful tool for enhancing energy, protecting cells, and improving overall health. To understand its effects, we need to first revisit the mitochondria—the engines of your cells.

The Foundation: Mitochondria and Energy Production

Mitochondria are responsible for generating energy in the form of ATP (adenosine triphosphate), which powers everything your body does. This energy production happens through a process called the electron transport chain (ETC).

Picture the ETC as a factory assembly line. Food is broken down into molecules that are passed along this chain, where electrons are transferred step by step, creating energy. However, this process isn't always perfect. Stress, aging, and damage can cause "bottlenecks" in the chain, reducing energy output and generating harmful byproducts like free radicals. When this happens, cells struggle to function, leading to fatigue, brain fog, and even chronic diseases.

Methylene Blue as a Mitochondrial Enhancer

Methylene blue directly interacts with the mitochondria to optimize energy production.

Here's how it works, step by step:

1. **Acts as an Electron Donor:** Methylene blue can donate electrons, effectively "jump-starting" the electron transport chain when it's stalled. Think of it as a helper that bridges broken links in the chain, keeping the energy assembly line running smoothly. This ensures your cells can produce more ATP, which translates to increased energy for your body and brain.

2. **Improves Oxygen Efficiency:** In situations where oxygen levels are low—like during stress, illness, or aging—mitochondria can struggle to produce energy. Methylene blue helps by facilitating better oxygen utilization, ensuring that energy production continues even when conditions aren't ideal.

3. **Reduces Energy Waste:** Inefficient mitochondria can waste energy and produce excessive free radicals, which damage cells and contribute to aging. Methylene blue improves mitochondrial efficiency, reducing these harmful byproducts while enhancing energy output.

Methylene Blue as an Antioxidant

Beyond its role in energy production, methylene blue is also a powerful **antioxidant**, protecting cells from oxidative stress. Oxidative stress occurs when free radicals—unstable molecules produced during energy production—outnumber the body's ability to neutralize them. Over time, this imbalance can damage mitochondria, DNA, and other vital cell components.

Methylene blue helps in two critical ways:

1. **Neutralizes Free Radicals:** It scavenges harmful molecules before they can cause damage, protecting your mitochondria and ensuring they function optimally.

2. **Prevents Cellular Damage:** By reducing oxidative stress, methylene blue slows aging at the cellular level, supporting long-term health and resilience.

Why This Matters to You

Methylene blue's unique mechanisms of action—boosting mitochondrial function, enhancing oxygen utilization, and neutralizing oxidative stress—address the root causes of fatigue, cognitive decline, and cellular aging. It's not a surface-level fix but a deep, foundational solution that supports your body's ability to thrive. Whether you're looking to boost energy, sharpen focus, or promote longevity, methylene blue provides a scientifically validated way to enhance your body's most vital systems. By understanding these mechanisms, you can better appreciate why methylene blue is a cornerstone of modern health and biohacking.

THE ANTIOXIDANT POWER OF METHYLENE BLUE

Every second, your cells are engaged in the vital process of energy production, powered by mitochondria—the tiny engines that fuel your body and mind. But this process comes with a downside: it generates free radicals, unstable molecules that can damage your cells. Left unchecked, free radicals lead to oxidative stress, a major driver of aging, fatigue, and chronic diseases. Here's where methylene blue shines as a potent antioxidant, offering protection and repair at the cellular level.

Understanding Oxidative Stress

To appreciate the antioxidant power of methylene blue, let's first explore oxidative stress. During energy production in mitochondria, electrons sometimes "leak" from the electron transport chain. These stray electrons interact with oxygen, creating free radicals. While your body has natural defenses—like enzymes and antioxidants—to neutralize these molecules, they can become overwhelmed by factors like stress, pollution, and aging.

When free radicals accumulate, they damage essential cellular components, including:

- **Mitochondria:** Impaired energy production.
- **DNA:** Genetic mutations and aging.
- **Cell Membranes:** Reduced cell function and increased vulnerability to disease.

This cumulative damage contributes to fatigue, cognitive decline, and visible aging. Controlling oxidative stress is essential for maintaining health and vitality.

How Methylene Blue Acts as an Antioxidant

Methylene blue is a unique and powerful antioxidant that works at the mitochondrial level to protect and repair cells. Unlike many antioxidants, which only work in specific areas of the cell, methylene blue operates directly within mitochondria, where oxidative stress is most concentrated.

Here's how it works:

1. **Neutralizing Free Radicals:** Methylene blue has a remarkable ability to "donate" electrons, stabilizing free radicals before they can cause damage. Imagine a firefighter putting out a spark before it becomes a blaze. This proactive approach protects mitochondria and other cellular structures from harm.

2. **Recycling Itself:** Unlike many antioxidants that are used up after neutralizing a free radical, methylene blue can regenerate itself. This recycling ability means it provides ongoing protection, making it highly efficient at reducing oxidative stress over time.

3. **Preventing Chain Reactions:** Free radicals can trigger chain reactions that damage multiple molecules in succession. Methylene blue interrupts these chains, minimizing the overall impact of oxidative stress on your cells.

Supporting Cellular Repair

Cellular repair is essential for maintaining health and reversing damage caused by stress, aging, and toxins. Methylene blue excels in this area, working on multiple levels to restore and protect your cells. By targeting key structures like mitochondria, DNA, and cell membranes, methylene blue supports robust cellular recovery and resilience. Here's how it works:

1. **Mitochondrial Recovery:** Mitochondria are the power plants of your cells, generating the energy needed for repair and survival. When mitochondria are damaged, energy production falters, leading to cellular dysfunction. Methylene blue protects and stabilizes mitochondria, ensuring efficient energy production. By optimizing this vital process, it restores cellular function and boosts resilience, giving your cells the resources they need to repair themselves effectively.

2. **DNA Integrity:** DNA is your cell's blueprint, essential for proper function and replication. Damage to DNA can lead to mutations, aging, and chronic diseases. Methylene blue safeguards your genetic material by neutralizing oxidative stress and promoting repair processes. This protection supports healthy aging and reduces the risk of long-term cellular damage.

3. **Membrane Stability:** Cell membranes act as the gatekeepers of the cell, regulating communication and nutrient flow. Methylene blue strengthens these membranes, enhancing their stability and functionality. This improved membrane health fosters better communication between cells and ensures a supportive environment for recovery.

The Benefits for You

The antioxidant power of methylene blue translates into tangible health benefits:

- **Increased Energy:** By reducing oxidative stress, methylene blue ensures that mitochondria can function efficiently, providing sustained energy.
- **Cognitive Clarity:** Protecting brain cells from oxidative damage sharpens focus, memory, and mental performance.
- **Anti-Aging:** Slowing oxidative damage at the cellular level reduces visible signs of aging and promotes longevity.
- **Enhanced Recovery:** Whether from exercise, illness, or stress, methylene blue helps your cells bounce back faster.

Why Methylene Blue Stands Out

Unlike generic antioxidants, methylene blue works directly at the source of oxidative stress—your mitochondria. Its dual role as an antioxidant and a mitochondrial enhancer makes it a cornerstone for optimizing health. By protecting your cells from damage and supporting their repair, methylene blue helps you feel and perform your best, every day. Understanding its antioxidant power reveals why it's an indispensable tool in the quest for vitality and longevity.

CHAPTER 3: THE PROVEN HEALTH BENEFITS OF METHYLENE BLUE

Methylene blue is more than just a scientifically intriguing compound—it's a tool with real, life-changing benefits. By optimizing mitochondrial function, reducing oxidative stress, and enhancing cellular health, it addresses many of the root causes of energy depletion, cognitive decline, aging, and illness. In this chapter, we'll explore six major ways methylene blue can transform your health and well-being.

BOOSTING ENERGY AND COMBATING FATIGUE

Fatigue is one of the most common challenges in modern life. Whether it's caused by a demanding schedule, lack of sleep, stress, or chronic health conditions, persistent low energy can feel like an insurmountable barrier to living fully. At its core, fatigue often stems from mitochondrial dysfunction—when the "power plants" of your cells fail to produce enough energy. Methylene blue stands out as a powerful tool to combat fatigue by directly enhancing mitochondrial function and improving energy production.

Understanding Energy Production and Mitochondrial Health

To grasp how methylene blue boosts energy, it's essential to understand the role of mitochondria. These tiny organelles are responsible for producing ATP (adenosine triphosphate), the molecule that fuels nearly all bodily functions. The process of generating ATP occurs through a series of steps called the electron transport chain (ETC). However, stress, toxins, aging, and chronic illnesses can disrupt the ETC, leading to reduced ATP production. When mitochondria falter, your cells don't get the energy they need, resulting in fatigue, sluggishness, and brain fog.

How Methylene Blue Restores Energy

Methylene blue supports your mitochondria in multiple ways, making it highly effective at fighting fatigue:

- **Acts as an Electron Donor:** In a healthy ETC, electrons flow smoothly through various proteins to generate ATP. But when this process stalls, energy production slows. Methylene blue steps in as an electron donor, bridging gaps in the chain and ensuring the process continues efficiently. Think of it as a jumper cable that gets your cellular engines running again.
- **Enhances Oxygen Utilization:** Oxygen is critical for ATP production, but when mitochondria are stressed, they can't use oxygen effectively. Methylene blue optimizes oxygen utilization, allowing your cells to produce energy even under challenging conditions, such as illness or low oxygen levels.

- **Reduces Energy Waste:** Inefficient mitochondria can waste energy and produce harmful byproducts like free radicals. Methylene blue improves mitochondrial efficiency, ensuring that more ATP is produced while minimizing energy waste.

Real-World Benefits

The practical benefits of methylene blue's energy-enhancing properties are profound:

- **Overcoming Chronic Fatigue:** Many individuals with conditions like chronic fatigue syndrome (CFS) or fibromyalgia have found methylene blue to be a game-changer. By restoring mitochondrial function, it helps alleviate the persistent exhaustion that defines these conditions.
- **Sustained Energy Throughout the Day:** Unlike stimulants that provide temporary boosts followed by crashes, methylene blue offers consistent energy by addressing the root cause of fatigue—poor mitochondrial health.
- **Improved Productivity and Focus:** For busy professionals, methylene blue's energy-boosting effects translate to better focus and efficiency, helping you power through demanding workdays without feeling drained.

Evidence Supporting Methylene Blue's Role

Scientific studies back methylene blue's ability to enhance energy production. Research has demonstrated its effectiveness in improving mitochondrial efficiency and reducing fatigue in animal and human models. Its unique ability to restore ATP production makes it a promising solution for individuals struggling with low energy.

Empowering Your Energy Transformation

Imagine waking up each day with sustained energy, mental clarity, and the drive to tackle anything life throws at you. Methylene blue offers this possibility by targeting the root cause of fatigue at the cellular level. With its scientifically proven ability to enhance mitochondrial function, methylene blue empowers you to reclaim your energy and vitality—naturally and effectively.

ENHANCING COGNITIVE PERFORMANCE AND MENTAL CLARITY

Mental clarity and cognitive performance are crucial for excelling in today's fast-paced world. Whether you're juggling work, family, or personal goals, staying focused and mentally sharp can feel like a constant challenge. Many factors—stress, aging, lack of sleep, or mitochondrial dysfunction—can contribute to brain fog and reduced cognitive function. Methylene blue offers a powerful solution, targeting the root causes of cognitive decline and enhancing your brain's performance at a cellular level.

The Brain's Energy Demands

Your brain is an energy-intensive organ, consuming up to 20% of your body's energy despite making up only about 2% of your weight.

This energy fuels essential processes like thinking, memory, focus, and problem-solving. The mitochondria in your brain cells play a critical role in producing ATP, the energy molecule that powers these functions. However, when mitochondrial efficiency declines—due to oxidative stress, aging, or illness—so does cognitive performance. The result is brain fog, difficulty concentrating, and slower mental processing.

How Methylene Blue Enhances Brain Function

Methylene blue supports cognitive performance by directly improving mitochondrial function and protecting brain cells.

Here's how it works:

1. **Optimizes Mitochondrial Efficiency:** Methylene blue acts as an electron donor, ensuring the mitochondria in your brain cells produce ATP more efficiently. By keeping the energy-production process running smoothly, methylene blue provides your brain with the energy it needs to maintain mental clarity and focus.

2. **Improves Oxygen Utilization:** Oxygen is essential for brain function, and methylene blue enhances its use in brain cells, ensuring consistent energy supply even under stress. This improved oxygen utilization helps maintain focus and sharp thinking, even during demanding tasks.

3. **Reduces Oxidative Stress:** The brain is especially vulnerable to oxidative stress, which can damage neurons and impair communication between brain cells. Methylene blue's antioxidant properties neutralize free radicals, protecting neurons from damage and preserving cognitive function.

4. **Promotes Neuroprotection:** Beyond energy production, methylene blue supports the brain's natural repair mechanisms. It reduces inflammation and prevents protein misfolding, which is linked to neurodegenerative diseases. This neuroprotective effect ensures long-term cognitive health.

Real-World Benefits

The cognitive benefits of methylene blue are both immediate and long-term:

- **Sharper Focus and Memory:** Many users report feeling more focused, alert, and mentally clear shortly after taking methylene blue. It's particularly helpful for professionals, students, or anyone working on mentally demanding tasks.
- **Improved Problem-Solving and Creativity:** By enhancing energy production and reducing oxidative stress, methylene blue supports the higher-order thinking required for solving complex problems and generating innovative ideas.
- **Reduced Brain Fog:** If you've ever struggled with mental sluggishness, methylene blue offers a solution by restoring mitochondrial function and providing the energy your brain needs to perform at its best.

Evidence Supporting Cognitive Benefits

Research demonstrates methylene blue's potential to enhance cognitive performance. Studies in humans and animals show improved memory, attention, and overall brain function after supplementation. For example, methylene blue has been investigated for its ability to improve memory recall and reduce cognitive decline in aging populations.

Reclaim Your Mental Edge

Imagine a life where your mind feels clear, your focus is sharp, and your mental performance is at its peak. Methylene blue provides the tools to achieve this by targeting the root causes of cognitive decline and restoring your brain's natural energy and resilience. With consistent use, methylene blue can empower you to think faster, focus better, and maintain clarity in every aspect of your life.

PROTECTING AGAINST NEURODEGENERATIVE DISEASES

Neurodegenerative diseases such as Alzheimer's, Parkinson's, and Huntington's disease are among the most feared health challenges, affecting millions worldwide. These conditions are often linked to the progressive decline of brain cells, driven by oxidative stress, mitochondrial dysfunction, and protein misfolding. While modern medicine offers few solutions to reverse these conditions, methylene blue has emerged as a promising tool to protect against and potentially slow the progression of neurodegenerative diseases. Its ability to support brain health at the cellular level makes it a powerful ally in preserving cognitive function.

Understanding Neurodegenerative Diseases

Neurodegenerative diseases occur when brain cells, or neurons, are damaged faster than they can be repaired or replaced.

This damage is typically caused by three interconnected factors:

1. **Mitochondrial Dysfunction:** When mitochondria fail to produce enough energy, neurons—high-energy cells—cannot perform their functions properly, leading to cognitive decline.
2. **Oxidative Stress:** Free radicals created during energy production can damage neurons, causing inflammation and accelerating cell death.
3. **Protein Misfolding:** Abnormal proteins, like beta-amyloid plaques in Alzheimer's or alpha-synuclein in Parkinson's, disrupt brain cell communication and trigger further degeneration.

How Methylene Blue Protects the Brain

Methylene blue addresses these root causes in several powerful ways:

1. **Enhances Mitochondrial Function:** Neurons rely heavily on mitochondria for energy. Methylene blue acts as an electron donor, restoring mitochondrial efficiency and ensuring that brain cells have the ATP they need to function. By keeping the brain's energy supply steady, methylene blue helps maintain neuron vitality.

2. **Reduces Oxidative Stress:** The brain is especially vulnerable to oxidative stress, which damages neurons and accelerates neurodegeneration. Methylene blue neutralizes harmful free radicals, protecting neurons from oxidative damage. Think of it as a protective shield, keeping your brain cells safe from daily wear and tear.
3. **Prevents Protein Misfolding:** Protein misfolding is a hallmark of many neurodegenerative diseases. Methylene blue stabilizes these proteins, preventing them from clumping together and disrupting brain function. For example, research shows that methylene blue can reduce the buildup of tau proteins and beta-amyloid plaques associated with Alzheimer's disease.
4. **Promotes Neuroprotection:** Beyond prevention, methylene blue actively supports brain repair mechanisms. It reduces inflammation, enhances neuronal communication, and stimulates processes that help brain cells recover from damage.

Real-World Benefits

The neuroprotective effects of methylene blue translate into tangible benefits for your brain health:

- **Prevention of Cognitive Decline:** Regular use can help stave off memory loss and other early signs of neurodegeneration, allowing you to stay sharp as you age.
- **Support for At-Risk Individuals:** For those with a family history of Alzheimer's or Parkinson's, methylene blue offers a proactive way to protect against these conditions.
- **Improved Quality of Life:** Individuals already experiencing cognitive challenges may benefit from enhanced focus, memory, and mental clarity due to methylene blue's ability to stabilize and support brain function.

Evidence Supporting Methylene Blue's Role

Research underscores methylene blue's potential in neurodegenerative diseases. Studies have shown its ability to reduce tau protein aggregation in Alzheimer's models and improve mitochondrial function in Parkinson's disease. In clinical trials, methylene blue has demonstrated improvements in memory and cognitive performance for individuals with mild cognitive impairment.

Protect Your Brain for the Future

Imagine maintaining your mental sharpness and clarity well into old age, free from the fear of neurodegenerative diseases. Methylene blue offers a scientifically validated way to protect your brain at the cellular level. By addressing the root causes of neurodegeneration—mitochondrial dysfunction, oxidative stress, and protein misfolding—it empowers you to take control of your cognitive health and preserve your most vital asset: your mind.

ANTI-AGING AND LONGEVITY: SLOWING CELLULAR DECLINE

Aging is a natural process, but its effects—fatigue, wrinkles, slower recovery, and cognitive decline—don't have to dominate your life. At its core, aging is driven by cellular decline, where your body's ability to repair and regenerate diminishes over time.

Methylene blue offers a groundbreaking approach to slow this process by targeting the root causes of aging: oxidative stress, mitochondrial dysfunction, and cellular damage. By supporting these foundational systems, methylene blue empowers you to age gracefully and maintain vitality.

The Cellular Basis of Aging

Aging occurs because cells experience cumulative damage over time. Three main processes contribute to this decline:

1. **Oxidative Stress:** Free radicals, created during energy production, damage DNA, proteins, and cell membranes. This accelerates aging and promotes disease.
2. **Mitochondrial Dysfunction:** Over time, mitochondria become less efficient, reducing energy production and impairing cellular repair mechanisms.
3. **Cellular Senescence:** Aging cells stop dividing and release inflammatory signals, disrupting tissue function and contributing to visible signs of aging.

How Methylene Blue Slows Aging

Methylene blue combats cellular aging through several mechanisms:

- **Neutralizing Oxidative Stress:** Free radicals are a major driver of cellular aging, damaging vital components of cells. Methylene blue acts as a potent antioxidant, neutralizing free radicals and preventing this damage. Think of it as a shield that protects your cells from daily wear and tear, allowing them to function optimally for longer.
- **Restoring Mitochondrial Function:** Mitochondria are critical for energy production and cellular repair. Methylene blue enhances mitochondrial efficiency, ensuring a steady supply of ATP. By keeping these energy factories running smoothly, it slows the decline of energy-dependent processes like tissue regeneration and immune function.
- **Protecting DNA Integrity:** DNA damage accelerates aging by impairing cell function and triggering mutations. Methylene blue safeguards your genetic material by reducing oxidative stress and supporting DNA repair mechanisms. This protection is crucial for maintaining healthy cell division and reducing the risk of age-related diseases.
- **Improving Cellular Communication:** Aging cells often release inflammatory molecules, disrupting communication between cells and promoting systemic inflammation. Methylene blue stabilizes cell membranes and reduces inflammation, promoting harmony between cells and supporting tissue health.

Real-World Benefits of Slowing Aging

The anti-aging effects of methylene blue are both visible and internal:

- **Youthful Skin:** By reducing oxidative damage and promoting collagen production, methylene blue can improve skin elasticity and reduce wrinkles.
- **Sustained Energy:** Enhanced mitochondrial function leads to higher energy levels, even as you age.
- **Sharper Mind:** By protecting neurons and preventing cognitive decline, methylene blue supports mental clarity well into old age.

- **Longer Healthspan:** Beyond extending lifespan, methylene blue helps maintain a high quality of life by preserving physical and mental vitality.

Scientific Evidence

Studies have shown that methylene blue extends the lifespan of model organisms like worms and flies by reducing oxidative stress and preserving mitochondrial function. In human studies, its anti-aging properties have been linked to improved skin health, cognitive performance, and cellular resilience.

Empower Your Longevity Journey

Imagine a future where aging doesn't limit your potential—where you maintain your energy, clarity, and vitality at any age. Methylene blue offers a scientifically supported tool to achieve this by addressing the root causes of aging. With regular use, you can slow cellular decline, enhance your longevity, and continue thriving in every stage of life.

SUPPORTING IMMUNE HEALTH AND FIGHTING INFECTIONS

Your immune system is your body's defense against infections, toxins, and harmful pathogens. However, modern lifestyles, stress, and aging can weaken this crucial system, leaving you more vulnerable to illness. Methylene blue offers a unique approach to enhancing immune function and combating infections. By supporting cellular health, reducing inflammation, and directly targeting pathogens, it strengthens your immune defenses in a holistic and powerful way.

Strengthening Immune Cells

Your immune system relies on a network of cells—white blood cells, T-cells, and macrophages— to identify and neutralize harmful invaders. These cells are highly energy-dependent, requiring robust mitochondrial function to perform their tasks efficiently. Methylene blue plays a vital role by enhancing mitochondrial function in immune cells, ensuring they have the energy needed to patrol, respond, and repair.

- **Improved Energy for Immune Cells:** Methylene blue boosts ATP production, giving immune cells the power to detect and fight pathogens effectively.
- **Faster Immune Response:** With optimized energy, immune cells can respond more quickly to infections, reducing the severity and duration of illness.

Reducing Inflammation

Chronic inflammation weakens the immune system, making it harder for your body to fend off infections. Methylene blue combats this issue by reducing oxidative stress and stabilizing inflammatory signals.

- **Neutralizing Free Radicals:** During immune responses, free radicals are produced as a byproduct. While these molecules help fight infections, excess amounts can damage healthy cells and prolong inflammation. Methylene blue's antioxidant properties neutralize these free radicals, preventing collateral damage.

- **Calming Overactive Inflammation:** By modulating inflammatory cytokines, methylene blue helps balance the immune system, ensuring it's neither overreactive (causing autoimmune issues) nor underperforming.

Direct Antimicrobial Action

One of methylene blue's most unique qualities is its direct antimicrobial effect. It has been shown to kill bacteria, viruses, and even parasites by disrupting their metabolic processes.

Here's how it works:

- **Targeting Pathogen Mitochondria:** Just as methylene blue supports your mitochondria, it can disrupt the energy production of harmful microorganisms, making it harder for them to survive.
- **Photoactivation:** When exposed to light, methylene blue becomes even more potent, generating reactive oxygen species that destroy pathogens. This makes it particularly effective in photodynamic therapy for treating localized infections.

Historically, methylene blue was used to treat malaria and urinary tract infections, and modern research continues to explore its potential against antibiotic-resistant bacteria and emerging viral threats.

Real-World Benefits

The immune-boosting and antimicrobial effects of methylene blue translate into practical health benefits:

- **Fewer Infections:** Regular use can help prevent common illnesses like colds, flu, and urinary tract infections.
- **Faster Recovery:** By supporting immune efficiency, methylene blue shortens recovery time from infections.
- **Resilience to Stress:** Chronic stress weakens the immune system, but methylene blue's anti-inflammatory and energy-enhancing effects help bolster your defenses.

Evidence Supporting Immune Benefits

Research shows that methylene blue enhances immune cell function, reduces inflammatory damage, and fights infections at multiple levels. Its history of treating diseases like malaria highlights its antimicrobial effectiveness, while modern studies support its role in improving immune resilience.

Empower Your Immune Health

Imagine feeling confident in your body's ability to ward off illness and recover quickly when challenges arise. Methylene blue offers a scientifically backed way to support your immune system, strengthen your defenses, and fight infections naturally. By incorporating it into your wellness routine, you can empower your health and maintain resilience in today's demanding world.

IMPROVING PHYSICAL PERFORMANCE AND RECOVERY

Whether you're an athlete pushing your limits, a fitness enthusiast striving for new personal bests, or someone who simply wants to recover faster after physical activity, optimizing performance and recovery is crucial. Methylene blue is a unique tool in this quest, offering profound benefits for energy production, endurance, and recovery at the cellular level. By supporting mitochondria and reducing oxidative stress, methylene blue helps you perform better and bounce back faster.

Enhancing Energy for Physical Performance

Physical performance hinges on the ability of your muscles to produce energy efficiently. This energy is generated in mitochondria through a process called cellular respiration, where food and oxygen are converted into ATP, the molecule that powers muscle contractions. However, during intense exercise, mitochondria can struggle to keep up with demand, leading to fatigue.

Methylene blue optimizes mitochondrial function, ensuring a steady supply of ATP even under high stress.

Here's how:

- **Boosts Energy Production:** By acting as an electron donor, methylene blue keeps the electron transport chain running smoothly, maximizing ATP output during exercise.
- **Improves Oxygen Utilization:** It enhances the efficiency of oxygen use in mitochondria, allowing muscles to sustain activity for longer periods.

Real-World Impact: Imagine being able to push through an extra mile in your run or add a few more reps to your workout, thanks to the enhanced energy methylene blue provides.

Reducing Muscle Fatigue and Oxidative Stress

Intense physical activity generates free radicals as a byproduct of energy production. These unstable molecules can cause oxidative stress, damaging muscle cells and contributing to soreness and fatigue. If left unchecked, oxidative stress can hinder performance and delay recovery.

Methylene blue's antioxidant properties help:

- **Neutralize Free Radicals:** It scavenges harmful molecules, preventing cellular damage and preserving muscle function.
- **Protect Mitochondria:** By shielding mitochondria from oxidative stress, methylene blue ensures they remain efficient even after strenuous activity.

Real-World Impact: Athletes often notice reduced post-workout fatigue and soreness, enabling them to train harder and recover faster.

Accelerating Recovery

Recovery is as important as performance. During recovery, your body repairs micro-tears in muscle fibers, clears out metabolic waste, and replenishes energy stores. Methylene blue accelerates these processes by:

- **Supporting Cellular Repair:** It promotes mitochondrial recovery, ensuring cells have the energy needed for repair and regeneration.
- **Reducing Inflammation:** Intense exercise can trigger inflammation, slowing recovery. Methylene blue modulates inflammatory pathways, speeding up healing.

Real-World Impact: Faster recovery means you can maintain consistency in your training regimen, reducing downtime and maximizing progress.

Building Resilience Over Time

Regular use of methylene blue doesn't just improve performance and recovery in the short term—it builds resilience over time. By preserving mitochondrial function and reducing cumulative oxidative damage, it helps you sustain higher levels of physical activity for years to come.

Evidence Supporting Performance Benefits

Research demonstrates methylene blue's role in enhancing ATP production and reducing exercise-induced oxidative stress. Athletes and active individuals have reported improved stamina, faster recovery times, and reduced muscle soreness after incorporating methylene blue into their routines.

Empower Your Physical Potential

Imagine achieving your fitness goals with greater ease, feeling strong and energized during workouts, and recovering quickly afterward. Methylene blue offers a scientifically supported way to enhance your physical performance and resilience, empowering you to unlock your full potential in any physical pursuit. Whether you're training for a marathon or simply looking to feel your best, methylene blue can help you thrive.

CHAPTER 4: USING METHYLENE BLUE SAFELY AND EFFECTIVELY

Methylene blue is a powerful tool for enhancing health, but like any supplement or therapeutic, its benefits are maximized when used correctly and safely. This chapter provides a comprehensive guide on how to use methylene blue effectively, tailored to your goals, while addressing safety precautions and potential side effects. By the end, you'll feel confident in incorporating methylene blue into your wellness routine.

DOSAGE GUIDELINES FOR BEGINNERS AND ADVANCED USERS

Getting the dosage right is the key to unlocking the full potential of methylene blue. Whether you're just starting out or looking to maximize its benefits for advanced therapeutic goals, knowing how much to take and why is essential. This chapter breaks down exactly what you need to know—clear, practical guidelines tailored to your goals, from boosting energy to protecting your brain. With the right approach, methylene blue becomes a safe, effective tool to transform your health and well-being. Let's dive in and take the guesswork out of finding your ideal dose.

Start Low and Go Slow

For beginners, starting with a low dose is the safest way to introduce methylene blue into your routine. A gradual approach helps your body adjust and minimizes any potential side effects, such as mild nausea or blue-tinted urine.

- **Beginner Dosage:** Start with *0.5 mg per kilogram of body weight per day*. For example, if you weigh 70 kg (154 lbs), a beginner's dose would be approximately 35 mg daily.
- **How to Take It:** Begin with one dose in the morning, ideally with food or water, to improve absorption and reduce any stomach discomfort.

Adjusting Dosage for Your Goals

Once you've acclimated to a lower dose, you can adjust based on your specific health objectives:

1. **General Energy and Wellness:** A daily dose of *0.5–1 mg/kg* is sufficient to boost mitochondrial function, improve energy levels, and maintain overall cellular health.
2. **Cognitive Enhancement and Mental Clarity:** For sharper focus and better memory, a slightly higher dose of *0.5–1 mg/kg* can support brain function without overloading your system. Many users find this range effective for overcoming brain fog or increasing productivity.
3. **Neuroprotection and Advanced Therapeutic Use:** For individuals seeking to address conditions like neurodegeneration or chronic fatigue, doses up to *2–3 mg/kg daily* may be appropriate. However, higher doses should only be used under medical supervision to ensure safety.

4. **Short-Term Recovery or Acute Use:** For occasional recovery boosts after intense exercise or illness, a dose of *1 mg/kg* taken for a few days can enhance mitochondrial recovery and resilience.

Step 3: Split Doses for Consistency

For doses higher than *1 mg/kg*, consider splitting your intake into two smaller doses throughout the day—morning and afternoon. This helps maintain stable levels in your system and reduces the likelihood of side effects like mild headaches.

Recognizing Individual Variation

Everyone's body reacts differently to methylene blue. Factors like weight, metabolism, and health conditions can influence how much is needed to achieve results. Start with the lowest effective dose, and increase gradually as needed. Keep track of how you feel and adjust accordingly.

Monitoring and Safety

While methylene blue is generally safe, exceeding *3 mg/kg daily* may increase the risk of side effects, such as dizziness, nausea, or serotonin-related interactions. If you're unsure about dosing, consult a healthcare provider.

METHODS OF ADMINISTRATION: ORAL, SUBLINGUAL, TOPICAL, AND INTRAVENOUS

Methylene blue is a versatile compound, and one of its strengths is the variety of ways it can be administered. Each method offers unique benefits, and the choice often depends on your health goals, lifestyle, and level of experience. This section will guide you through the most common methods of administration—oral, sublingual, topical, and intravenous—so you can confidently choose the approach that works best for you.

Oral Administration

Taking methylene blue orally is the most common and straightforward method, making it ideal for beginners and general wellness goals.

- **How It Works:** The liquid or capsule form is swallowed and absorbed through the digestive system, delivering systemic effects throughout the body.
- **Best For:** Energy enhancement, neuroprotection, and cognitive support.
- **Pros:**
    1. Convenient and easy for daily use.
    2. Suitable for long-term health maintenance.
- **Cons:**
    1. Slower absorption compared to other methods.
    2. May cause temporary blue staining of the mouth, teeth, or tongue.
- **Practical Tips:** Mix methylene blue with water to dilute the taste and prevent staining. Rinse your mouth afterward to minimize discoloration.

Sublingual Administration

For faster absorption and a more immediate effect, sublingual administration is an excellent option.

- **How It Works:** Methylene blue is placed under the tongue, where it absorbs directly into the bloodstream, bypassing the digestive system.
- **Best For:** Rapid cognitive enhancement, focus, and short-term energy boosts.
- **Pros:**
    1. Faster onset of effects compared to oral administration.
    2. Avoids digestive breakdown, delivering a more potent dose.
- **Cons:**
    1. Slightly more effort than swallowing a capsule.
    2. Some users may experience mild irritation under the tongue.
- **Practical Tips:** Hold the liquid or tablet under your tongue for 1–2 minutes before swallowing. Avoid eating or drinking for a few minutes after to maximize absorption.

Topical Administration

Methylene blue can also be applied to the skin for localized benefits, making this method popular for cosmetic or dermatological uses.

- **How It Works:** The compound is diluted and applied to the skin, where it penetrates cells locally without entering the systemic circulation significantly.
- **Best For:** Improving skin health, enhancing elasticity, and treating minor wounds or inflammation.
- **Pros:**
    1. Targets specific areas directly.
    2. Reduces systemic exposure, minimizing potential side effects.
- **Cons:**
    1. Limited to localized benefits.
    2. May temporarily stain the skin blue.
- **Practical Tips:** Dilute methylene blue in a carrier oil or water before applying to the skin. Perform a patch test first to check for any sensitivity.

Intravenous (IV) Administration

Intravenous administration is the most potent and efficient way to deliver methylene blue, but it should only be performed by a medical professional.

- **How It Works:** Methylene blue is injected directly into the bloodstream, providing immediate and powerful effects.
- **Best For:** Acute conditions, advanced therapeutic needs, and severe mitochondrial dysfunction.
- **Pros:**
    1. Rapid and potent delivery of methylene blue.
    2. Directly supports systemic and cellular function.

- **Cons:**
    1. Requires professional administration.
    2. Higher risk of side effects like nausea or dizziness.
- **Practical Tips:** Only undergo IV administration under medical supervision. It's typically reserved for hospital settings or advanced clinical applications.

Choosing the Right Method

Selecting the best method for administering methylene blue depends on your health goals, lifestyle, and level of experience. Each method—oral, sublingual, topical, or intravenous—offers unique benefits.

Here's a step-by-step guide to help you decide which one is right for you:

Oral Administration:
- **Best for:** Beginners, general wellness, energy enhancement, and neuroprotection.
- **Why Choose It:** Oral administration is simple and effective for long-term daily use. By swallowing methylene blue in liquid or capsule form, you benefit from gradual absorption and systemic effects.
- **Consider This:** This method is slower-acting compared to sublingual or IV options, but it's a great starting point.

Sublingual Administration:
- **Best for:** Quick cognitive boosts, focus, and mental clarity.
- **Why Choose It:** Sublingual use bypasses digestion, delivering faster and more potent effects. Perfect for short-term performance enhancement.
- **Consider This:** It requires holding the dose under your tongue for a minute or two for optimal absorption.

Topical Application:
- **Best for:** Skin health, wound care, and localized benefits.
- **Why Choose It:** Applying methylene blue directly to the skin targets specific areas without systemic effects.

Intravenous (IV):
- **Best for:** Severe conditions and professional treatments.
- **Why Choose It:** IV administration is the most efficient but should only be performed under medical supervision.

Choose the method that fits your goals and start experiencing the benefits of methylene blue safely and effectively.

UNDERSTANDING AND MANAGING SIDE EFFECTS

Like any supplement or therapeutic compound, methylene blue can produce side effects, especially if taken at higher doses or without proper precautions. While most side effects are harmless and manageable, understanding them helps you use methylene blue safely and confidently. This section outlines common side effects, why they occur, and practical tips for minimizing or avoiding them.

Recognizing Common Side Effects

Using methylene blue is generally safe when following proper protocols, but like any supplement, it can have side effects. Most are mild, temporary, and easy to manage, especially if you're aware of what to expect. Let's explore the most common side effects, why they occur, and how to handle them with confidence.

1. **Blue or Green Urine and Stool**
    *   **What Happens:** After taking methylene blue, you may notice your urine or stool turning blue or green. This is one of the most noticeable side effects, and while surprising at first, it's completely harmless.
    *   **Why It Happens:** Methylene blue is highly pigmented, and your body excretes it naturally through urine and feces.
    *   **How to Manage It:** There's nothing to worry about—it's a normal process. Consider it a visual reminder that the compound is working in your system.

2. **Mild Nausea or Stomach Upset**
    *   **What Happens:** Some users experience slight nausea or discomfort in their stomach after taking methylene blue, especially when starting out.
    *   **Why It Happens:** Methylene blue can irritate the stomach lining if taken on an empty stomach or in high concentrations.
    *   **How to Manage It:** Take methylene blue with food or a full glass of water to reduce irritation. Starting with a low dose and gradually increasing can also help your body adapt.

3. **Headaches or Lightheadedness**
    *   **What Happens:** You might feel a mild headache or slight dizziness, especially if you're dehydrated or taking higher doses.
    *   **Why It Happens:** This is often due to your body adjusting to enhanced mitochondrial activity, which increases energy production.
    *   **How to Manage It:** Stay hydrated and ensure you're taking the appropriate dose for your weight and goals. If headaches persist, reduce the dose slightly until your body adjusts.

4. **Temporary Blue Staining of the Mouth or Skin**
    *   **What Happens:** If methylene blue comes into contact with your skin, teeth, or tongue, it may leave a temporary blue tint.
    *   **Why It Happens:** Methylene blue is a strong dye, so any spill or direct application may stain.
    *   **How to Manage It:** Use a straw for oral doses to minimize contact with teeth, and rinse your mouth after swallowing. For topical applications, dilute the solution and apply carefully to avoid spills.

These common side effects, while sometimes unexpected, are generally harmless and manageable. By understanding why they happen and taking simple precautions, you can confidently incorporate methylene blue into your routine without unnecessary worry.

Rare but Serious Side Effects

While methylene blue is generally safe when used correctly, it's essential to be aware of rare but potentially serious side effects. These are uncommon, often occurring only with improper dosing or in individuals with specific health conditions or medication interactions. Understanding these risks empowers you to use methylene blue safely and confidently. Here's a step-by-step breakdown of what to watch for and how to minimize these risks.

1. **Serotonin Syndrome**
   - **What It Is:** A rare but serious condition caused by excessive serotonin levels in the brain. It occurs when methylene blue is taken with medications that also increase serotonin, such as SSRIs (selective serotonin reuptake inhibitors), MAOIs (monoamine oxidase inhibitors), or certain antidepressants.
   - **Symptoms:** Signs include confusion, agitation, rapid heart rate, sweating, tremors, or muscle stiffness. In severe cases, it can lead to seizures or unconsciousness.
   - **How to Avoid It:**
     - Avoid combining methylene blue with serotonergic medications unless under close medical supervision.
     - Always consult a healthcare professional if you're on antidepressants or mood-stabilizing drugs before starting methylene blue.

2. **Allergic Reactions**
   - **What It Is:** Although rare, some individuals may experience an allergic reaction to methylene blue. This can range from mild skin irritation to more severe symptoms.
   - **Symptoms:** Look for hives, swelling (especially in the face or throat), difficulty breathing, or severe itching.
   - **How to Avoid It:**
     - If you're trying methylene blue for the first time, start with a very small test dose to check for sensitivity.
     - Discontinue use immediately if symptoms appear, and seek medical attention for severe reactions.

3. **Hemolytic Anemia in G6PD Deficiency**
   - **What It Is:** People with G6PD deficiency (a genetic enzyme disorder) are at risk of hemolytic anemia—a condition where red blood cells break down prematurely—if they take methylene blue.
   - **Symptoms:** Fatigue, pale skin, jaundice, or shortness of breath after taking methylene blue.
   - **How to Avoid It:**
     - If you suspect or know you have G6PD deficiency, avoid methylene blue entirely unless directed by a doctor.

4. **Kidney or Bladder Irritation**
   - **What It Is:** At higher doses, methylene blue may irritate the urinary system, especially in those with pre-existing kidney conditions.
   - **Symptoms:** Discomfort during urination or increased frequency.
   - **How to Avoid It:**
     - Stay within recommended dosages.
     - Ensure you're well-hydrated to support kidney function and reduce urinary concentration.

5. **When to Seek Medical Attention:** If you experience severe symptoms such as difficulty breathing, rapid heartbeat, extreme confusion, or persistent discomfort, stop using methylene blue and seek medical care immediately. These occurrences are rare but should be addressed promptly.

Practical Tips to Minimize Side Effects

Using methylene blue can be a game-changer for your health, but like any powerful tool, it's important to use it wisely. While most side effects are mild and manageable, understanding how to minimize them is key to a smooth and successful experience. This section gives you clear, actionable tips to avoid discomfort and get the most out of methylene blue, so you can focus on its incredible benefits with confidence and ease.

1. **Start with a Low Dose and Increase Gradually**
   - **Why It Helps:** Starting with a smaller dose allows your body to adapt to methylene blue, reducing the likelihood of side effects like nausea, headaches, or dizziness.
   - **How to Do It:** Begin with *0.5 mg per kilogram of body weight per day*. For example, if you weigh 70 kg (154 lbs), start with about 35 mg daily. After a week or two, you can slowly increase the dose if needed, based on your health goals and tolerance.

2. **Stay Well-Hydrated**
   - **Why It Helps:** Hydration supports kidney function, helping your body process and excrete methylene blue more effectively. This can reduce headaches, nausea, and potential urinary irritation.
   - **How to Do It:** Drink at least 8–10 glasses of water daily, particularly before and after taking methylene blue. Adding electrolytes can further support hydration and energy levels.

3. **Take It with Food**
   - **Why It Helps:** Taking methylene blue on an empty stomach can sometimes irritate the stomach lining, leading to mild nausea or discomfort.
   - **How to Do It:** Pair your dose with a meal or a snack, such as a piece of fruit, yogurt, or a protein-rich option. This can buffer your stomach and improve absorption.

4. **Avoid Mixing with Certain Medications**
   - **Why It Helps:** Some medications, particularly SSRIs and MAOIs, can interact with methylene blue, increasing the risk of serotonin syndrome.
   - **How to Do It:** If you are taking antidepressants or other medications, consult your heal-

thcare provider before starting methylene blue. This precaution helps you avoid harmful interactions.

5. **Use the Right Administration Method**
   - **Why It Helps:** Choosing the method of administration that suits your goals can reduce unnecessary side effects.
   - **How to Do It:** For general wellness, oral or sublingual methods are effective. If you're prone to nausea, consider sublingual use to bypass the digestive system. For skin health, use topical application to avoid systemic effects.

6. **Address Blue Staining**
   - Why It Helps: Methylene blue can temporarily stain your mouth, teeth, or skin, but this is easily manageable.
   - How to Do It: Use a straw for oral doses, rinse your mouth afterward, and apply topical methylene blue carefully to avoid spills.

Reassurance and Confidence

It's important to remember that most people tolerate methylene blue extremely well when using proper protocols. Side effects like blue urine or mild nausea may seem unusual but are manageable and usually temporary. By understanding these potential effects, you can approach methylene blue with confidence, knowing how to handle any minor discomforts that may arise.

WHO SHOULD AVOID METHYLENE BLUE: SAFETY PRECAUTIONS

While methylene blue is safe and effective for most people, there are specific circumstances where it should be used with caution or avoided altogether. Understanding these safety precautions is essential for ensuring that your experience with methylene blue is both positive and risk-free. In this section, we'll outline who should avoid methylene blue, when to consult a healthcare provider, and how to use it responsibly.

Individuals with G6PD Deficiency
- **What is G6PD Deficiency:** G6PD (glucose-6-phosphate dehydrogenase) deficiency is a genetic condition that affects red blood cell health. People with this condition are at risk of developing hemolytic anemia (a rapid breakdown of red blood cells) when exposed to certain substances, including methylene blue.
- **Why It Matters:** Methylene blue can trigger oxidative stress in red blood cells, leading to complications in those with G6PD deficiency.
- **Precaution:** If you suspect or know you have G6PD deficiency, avoid using methylene blue unless explicitly recommended by a doctor under close supervision.

Pregnant or Breastfeeding Women

- **Why It Matters:** The safety of methylene blue during pregnancy and breastfeeding has not been thoroughly studied. While it has been used in certain medical contexts during pregnancy, it's best to avoid it unless absolutely necessary and prescribed by a healthcare provider.
- **Precaution:** Pregnant or breastfeeding individuals should consult their doctor before considering methylene blue.

People Taking Certain Medications

Methylene blue interacts with specific medications, potentially leading to dangerous side effects. The most notable concern is serotonin syndrome, a condition caused by excess serotonin in the brain.

- **Medications to Avoid with Methylene Blue**
  1. **SSRIs (Selective Serotonin Reuptake Inhibitors):** Common antidepressants like fluoxetine, sertraline, and citalopram.
  2. **MAOIs (Monoamine Oxidase Inhibitors):** Another class of antidepressants that can increase serotonin levels.
  3. **Other Serotonergic Drugs:** Tramadol, certain migraine medications, and supplements like St. John's Wort.
- **Why It Matters:** Combining methylene blue with these drugs can increase serotonin levels to dangerous levels, causing confusion, agitation, rapid heart rate, and in severe cases, seizures.
- **Precaution:** If you're taking any of these medications, consult your healthcare provider before using methylene blue. Do not stop taking prescribed medications without medical advice.

Individuals with Kidney Disorders

- **Why It Matters:** Methylene blue is excreted through the kidneys, and those with kidney disease or compromised kidney function may have difficulty processing it. This could lead to an accumulation of the compound in the body, increasing the risk of side effects.
- **Precaution:** Speak with a healthcare provider if you have a history of kidney disease before starting methylene blue.

People with Severe Respiratory Conditions

- **Why It Matters:** Methylene blue can affect oxygen transport in the blood. While this is typically a non-issue for healthy individuals, those with severe respiratory disorders, such as COPD, may experience complications.
- **Precaution:** Use methylene blue cautiously and under medical supervision if you have a respiratory condition.

When in Doubt, Consult a Professional

For most individuals, methylene blue is safe when used properly. However, if you fall into any of the categories mentioned above or have a pre-existing medical condition, it's essential to consult a healthcare provider before starting methylene blue. This ensures that any risks are identified and managed appropriately.

CHAPTER 5: INTEGRATING METHYLENE BLUE INTO YOUR BIOHACKING ROUTINE

If you're serious about taking control of your energy, focus, and health, methylene blue can be a game-changer—but only if you know how to use it effectively. This chapter cuts through the guesswork and shows you exactly how to integrate methylene blue into your daily biohacking routine. You'll learn how to create a protocol that fits your specific goals, pair it with other proven tools like light therapy or NAD+ for even greater results, and track your progress so you can see the transformation unfold. Biohacking isn't just about experimenting—it's about measurable success, and methylene blue can help you get there faster. Let's get started.

CREATING A PERSONALIZED PROTOCOL FOR ENERGY, COGNITION, AND WELLNESS

Integrating methylene blue into your daily routine starts with understanding your personal biohacking goals. Whether you want more energy to power through the day, enhanced mental clarity to stay sharp, or overall wellness and longevity, creating a tailored protocol is key to success. This section will walk you step by step through building a plan that fits seamlessly into your life.

Step 1: Define Your Biohacking Goals

Before you start, ask yourself: **What do I want to achieve?** Your goals will determine your dosage, timing, and methods of administration.

1. **For Energy and Fatigue Relief:** If you struggle with afternoon slumps or low energy levels, focus on morning dosing to jumpstart your day and provide sustained energy.
2. **For Cognitive Performance:** If your goal is sharper focus, improved memory, or tackling mentally demanding tasks, sublingual dosing just before a work session or important meeting can provide quick and noticeable results.
3. **For Overall Wellness and Longevity:** If your goal is cellular health, anti-aging, or general wellness, consistent daily use at lower doses is best.

Write down your main goals—this clarity will help you design a protocol that aligns with your needs.

Step 2: Choose the Right Dosage

The right dosage ensures effectiveness while minimizing side effects. Here's how to approach it:

- **Beginners:** Start with a low dose of *0.5 mg/kg body weight per day*. For example, if you weigh 70 kg (154 lbs), your starting dose would be approximately 35 mg. This helps your body adjust.
- **Energy and Cognition:** For boosting energy and mental clarity, aim for *0.5–1 mg/kg daily*.
- **Advanced Protocols:** For neuroprotection, longevity, or chronic fatigue, dosages of up to *2 mg/kg daily* may be considered, but only under medical supervision.

TIP: Start low, monitor your results, and increase gradually if needed.

Step 3: Time Your Doses for Maximum Impact

When you take methylene blue can significantly impact its benefits. Here's how to time your doses:

- **Morning:** Taking methylene blue in the morning helps improve energy, focus, and productivity throughout the day. Pair it with light exercise or a high-protein breakfast for enhanced effects.
- **Pre-Work or Study Sessions:** Use sublingual methylene blue 15–30 minutes before mentally demanding tasks for quick cognitive enhancement.
- **During Intermittent** Fasting: If you fast, methylene blue can provide an energy boost and mental clarity without breaking your fast.

Consistency is key—take methylene blue at the same time each day for best results.

Step 4: Combine Methylene Blue with Synergistic Biohacks

To amplify methylene blue's effects, pair it with complementary tools:

- **Red Light Therapy:** Use red or near-infrared light therapy after taking methylene blue to further stimulate mitochondrial energy production.
- **NAD+ Supplementation:** Stack methylene blue with NAD+ for enhanced cellular repair and anti-aging benefits.
- **Cold Therapy:** Pairing methylene blue with cold exposure boosts mitochondrial resilience and recovery.

These biohacks work together to elevate energy, improve cellular function, and accelerate results.

Step 5: Track Your Progress

To ensure your protocol is effective, track measurable changes. Use these metrics:

- **Energy Levels:** Monitor how you feel throughout the day. Are your afternoon slumps improving?
- **Mental Clarity:** Note improvements in focus, productivity, or memory.
- **Performance Benchmarks:** Track physical or mental tasks, such as exercise performance, work efficiency, or problem-solving speed.

Keep a daily journal to record your progress, including the dosage, timing, and any biohacks you paired with methylene blue.

Creating a personalized protocol is about experimentation, consistency, and listening to your body. Start small, track your results, and refine your approach to align with your goals. With methylene blue as a cornerstone of your biohacking journey, you can unlock higher energy, sharper focus, and long-term wellness, making every day an opportunity to optimize and thrive.

COMBINING METHYLENE BLUE WITH OTHER BIOHACKS: LIGHT THERAPY, NAD+, AND MORE

Methylene blue is impressive on its own, but when combined with other biohacks, it becomes a game-changer. Think of it as the centerpiece of your biohacking toolkit—ready to work even harder when paired with proven strategies like red light therapy, NAD+ supplementation, intermittent fasting, and cold exposure. In this section, you'll learn how to stack methylene blue with these tools to unlock higher energy, sharper focus, faster recovery, and enhanced longevity. This is where the magic happens—small, intentional combinations that deliver big, measurable results. Let's dive in and build your ultimate performance protocol.

Pairing Methylene Blue with Red Light Therapy

Red and near-infrared light therapy (photobiomodulation) enhances mitochondrial energy production by stimulating cytochrome c oxidase, a key enzyme in the electron transport chain. Methylene blue works on the same pathway, acting as an electron donor to optimize ATP production. When combined, these two biohacks amplify each other's effects.

- **How to Combine**
    1. Take your dose of methylene blue 15–30 minutes before a red light therapy session.
    2. Use red or near-infrared light (wavelengths between 600–850 nm) for 10–20 minutes, targeting your face, chest, or other areas needing recovery or energy boosts.
- **Benefits:** Increased energy production, faster recovery, improved cognitive function, and enhanced cellular repair.
- **Example:** If you're preparing for a mentally demanding day, take methylene blue sublingually in the morning and follow with a quick red light therapy session. You'll notice a sharp boost in focus and energy.

Combining Methylene Blue with NAD+ Supplementation

NAD+ (nicotinamide adenine dinucleotide) is a coenzyme essential for mitochondrial repair and energy production. Levels naturally decline with age, leading to fatigue, cellular damage, and aging. Methylene blue supports mitochondria by improving ATP production and reducing oxidative stress, while NAD+ enhances cellular repair processes.

- **How to Combine**
    1. Supplement with NAD+ precursors like nicotinamide riboside (NR) or nicotinamide mononucleotide (NMN) in the morning.
    2. Take methylene blue alongside NAD+ supplementation to optimize mitochondrial health and energy output.
- **Benefits:** Enhanced energy, improved cellular repair, anti-aging effects, and reduced brain fog.
- **Example:** Pairing methylene blue with NAD+ is ideal for individuals focused on longevity and neuroprotection. Use this combination daily as part of your morning wellness routine.

Integrating Methylene Blue with Intermittent Fasting

Intermittent fasting enhances mitochondrial efficiency, promotes autophagy (cellular clean-up), and improves focus by stabilizing blood sugar. Methylene blue further supports mitochondrial function during fasting, providing energy without breaking the fast.

- **How to Combine**
    1. Take methylene blue in the morning during your fasting window. Sublingual dosing is especially effective for quick energy and focus.
    2. Pair methylene blue with hydration and electrolytes to support energy levels during fasting.
- **Benefits:** Sustained energy, sharper focus during fasting periods, improved metabolic health, and cellular repair.
- **Example:** If you fast until noon, take methylene blue at 9 a.m. to maintain mental clarity and energy while extending the benefits of fasting.

Enhancing Resilience with Cold Exposure

Cold exposure (e.g., cold showers or cryotherapy) stimulates mitochondrial biogenesis, boosts metabolism, and reduces inflammation. Combined with methylene blue, it strengthens mitochondrial function and improves recovery.

- **How to Combine**
    1. Take methylene blue 15–30 minutes before cold exposure.
    2. Follow with 2–5 minutes of cold exposure (shower, ice bath, or cryotherapy).
- **Benefits:** Enhanced energy, increased metabolic resilience, faster muscle recovery, and reduced inflammation.
- **Example:** After a workout, take methylene blue, then use cold therapy to accelerate recovery and reduce soreness.

Building Your Biohacking Stack

Combining methylene blue with other biohacks can transform your health and performance.

Here's a sample morning routine:

1. **Wake Up:** Take methylene blue sublingually to jumpstart mitochondrial energy.
2. **Red Light Therapy:** Follow with a 10-minute red light session for enhanced ATP production.

3. **NAD+ Supplementation:** Add NAD+ precursors for cellular repair and anti-aging.
4. **Intermittent Fasting:** Extend your fast until noon for mental clarity and metabolic benefits.
5. **Cold Shower*:** Finish with 2 minutes of cold exposure to build resilience and reduce inflammation.

Combining methylene blue with other proven biohacks can supercharge your results. Whether you're seeking more energy, sharper focus, or better recovery, these tools work together to amplify each other's benefits. Start with one or two combinations, track your progress, and refine your protocol as you go. With consistency and creativity, methylene blue can become the cornerstone of a powerful and rewarding biohacking routine.

*Cold Shower

I completely understand—just the thought of taking a cold shower can feel unappealing. I felt the same way when my meditation and fitness instructor first suggested it to me. I used to take hot showers even in the middle of August because, for me, it was the ultimate way to relax. But I wanted to challenge myself and step out of my comfort zone. I'll admit, I was skeptical—I wouldn't have bet a dollar that I could last more than 5 seconds under cold water!

The key is, you can't jump straight from a "normal" shower to an ice-cold one; that's a recipe for failure. There's a method to doing it gradually and, believe it or not, you can still enjoy the experience without losing the comfort of your shower. Here's a step-by-step guide to help you ease into cold showers successfully—trust me, it's easier than you think!

Day 1: Start with the Legs (Knees Down)
1. Warm Start: Begin with your usual warm shower.
2. Lower Body Only:
   - Turn the water to cool (not cold) for the final 15-30 seconds.
   - Let the cool water flow over your legs below the knees.
3. Focus on Breathing: Practice slow, deep breathing to calm your body.

Day 2: Entire Legs
1. Warm Beginning: Start with warm water.
2. Extend the Cool Water to the Entire Legs:
   - Turn the temperature to cool for 30-45 seconds.
   - Let the cool water flow over your legs from the thighs down.
3. Stay Calm: Keep breathing deeply and remind yourself that this is manageable.

Day 3: Add the Belly and Lower Back
1. Warm Start: Start with a warm shower.
2. Legs and Midsection:
   - Switch to cool water for 45 seconds.
   - First, let it hit your legs as before.
   - Slowly bring the cool water up to your belly and lower back.
3. Breathing Tip: When exposing your midsection, take longer exhales to relax.

Day 4: Add the Chest and Shoulders

1. Warm Start: Begin as usual with warm water.
2. Legs and Upper Body:
   - Reduce the temperature to cool for 1 minute.
   - Let the water flow over your legs, belly, lower back, and now your chest and shoulders.
   - Spend about 15-20 seconds focusing on each area.
3. Stay Calm: As the water hits your chest, focus on maintaining controlled breathing.

Day 5: Full Body (Cool Water)

1. Warm Start: Start with warm water for comfort.
2. Full Body Exposure:
   - Turn the water to cool for 1-2 minutes.
   - Allow the water to hit your entire body, starting from your legs and gradually moving up to your torso, arms, and shoulders.
3. Mindset: Visualize the cool water as refreshing and energizing.

Day 6: Move to Cold Water (Full Body)

1. Warm Start (Optional): Start with warm water if needed.
2. Cold Exposure:
   - Switch to cold water for 1-2 minutes.
   - Allow the water to flow over your entire body as before.
3. Focus on Relaxing: Use deep, slow breaths to adapt to the shock.

Day 7: Full Cold Shower

1. Go Straight to Cold: Start your shower with cold water.
2. Full Body: Let the cold water hit your entire body for 1-2 minutes.
3. Embrace It: Focus on how invigorated and energized you feel after the cold exposure.

Key Tips for Success:

- **Deep Breathing:** Practice deep, steady breaths during cold exposure to help your body adapt and remain calm.
- **Positive Visualization:** Visualize yourself successfully completing each step to boost confidence and reduce discomfort.
- **Consistency:** Aim to practice this routine daily to help your body adjust more effectively.
- **Listen to Your Body:** If you experience significant discomfort or feel unwell, revert to a more comfortable temperature and consult a healthcare professional if necessary.

TRACKING PROGRESS AND MEASURING SUCCESS

Integrating methylene blue into your biohacking routine is only the first step. To truly unlock its potential, you need to track your progress and measure success. Biohacking is about achieving measurable, tangible improvements, and knowing what's working allows you to fine-tune your protocol for the best results. Whether your goal is boosting energy, sharpening mental focus, or supporting overall wellness, consistent tracking will help you stay motivated and maximize benefits. Here's a detailed, step-by-step guide to tracking your journey.

Define What Success Looks Like for You

Before you start tracking, it's essential to define your biohacking goals clearly. Ask yourself:

WHAT AM I TRYING TO IMPROVE
- Is it more energy throughout the day?
- Sharper focus and less brain fog?
- Faster recovery from workouts or reduced fatigue?
- Long-term wellness and anti-aging benefits?

Be specific with your goals. For example, instead of saying "I want more energy," aim for "I want to eliminate my afternoon slump and feel focused between 2–5 p.m." Clear goals give you benchmarks to measure success.

Choose Your Metrics

To measure progress effectively, select key metrics that align with your goals.

Here are some examples:

ENERGY LEVELS:
- Use a daily energy log or rating system (1–10) to monitor your energy throughout the day.
- Note when you feel most energized and when fatigue kicks in. This will help you identify patterns and the impact of methylene blue.

COGNITIVE PERFORMANCE:
Track focus, memory, and mental clarity using simple tools:
- Timed mental tasks like puzzles, reading comprehension, or brain-training apps (e.g., Lumosity, BrainHQ).
- Work productivity: Record how much you accomplish during key focus periods.
- Use journal entries to note improvements in concentration and creativity.

PHYSICAL PERFORMANCE AND RECOVERY:
- Track workout performance, such as stamina, endurance, or weightlifting progress.
- Note how quickly you recover after exercise and whether soreness or fatigue decreases.

GENERAL WELLNESS AND MOOD:
- Use a mood tracker or journal to note shifts in how you feel mentally and emotionally.
- Record improvements in sleep quality, stress levels, or overall well-being.

Use Tools to Track Data

To make tracking easier, incorporate tools and technology:

- **Journals and Logs:** Keep a daily notebook to track methylene blue use, dosage, timing, and effects.
- **Wearables:** Use devices like fitness trackers (Oura Ring, WHOOP, or Apple Watch) to monitor metrics like heart rate variability (HRV), sleep quality, and activity levels.
- **Mobile Apps:** Apps like Habit Tracker, Notion, or brain-training platforms help you log progress consistently.

Pairing methylene blue usage with measurable data ensures you can see the impact clearly.

Review and Adjust Regularly

Set aside time once a week or month to review your progress. Ask yourself:

- What's working well? Am I noticing more energy, sharper focus, or faster recovery?
- What could be improved? Do I need to adjust my dosage, timing, or stack methylene blue with other biohacks like light therapy?

Use your insights to refine your protocol, making small tweaks as needed. Remember, biohacking is an ongoing process of discovery.

Celebrate Your Wins

As you track progress, don't overlook the small victories. Whether it's finishing tasks more efficiently, waking up energized, or recovering faster from workouts, acknowledge these improvements. Success fuels momentum, and celebrating milestones keeps you motivated on your biohacking journey.

CHAPTER 6: ADVANCED APPLICATIONS OF METHYLENE BLUE

Methylene blue is breaking new ground in health and medicine. Beyond boosting energy and focus, it's showing incredible potential for tackling serious challenges like depression, PTSD, skin aging, and even cancer support. This chapter reveals how methylene blue is being used in advanced therapies, backed by emerging research and real-world results. If you're curious about how this remarkable compound can help with mental health, improve skin vitality, or support recovery from chronic conditions, you're about to discover its full potential. Let's explore the innovative ways methylene blue is transforming health care and offering new hope.

METHYLENE BLUE IN NEUROTHERAPY: DEPRESSION, ANXIETY, AND PTSD

Mental health disorders like depression, anxiety, and PTSD (Post-Traumatic Stress Disorder) are growing challenges worldwide. While traditional treatments like medication and therapy have helped many, there's a growing need for solutions that target the root causes of these conditions. Methylene blue, once primarily known as a medical dye and antimicrobial agent, is now emerging as a powerful tool in neurotherapy—offering hope to individuals struggling with mood disorders and trauma.

Here's a step-by-step explanation of how methylene blue works and why it's gaining recognition as a promising therapy for mental health.

The Link Between Brain Energy and Mental Health

Your brain is one of the most energy-hungry organs in your body, relying heavily on efficient mitochondrial function to produce energy (ATP) for cognitive and emotional processes.

In mental health disorders, studies have shown that:

- Mitochondrial dysfunction leads to reduced energy in brain cells.
- Oxidative stress causes inflammation, which can damage neurons and disrupt neurotransmitter balance.
- These issues contribute to symptoms like fatigue, brain fog, mood instability, and emotional distress.

Methylene blue addresses these root causes by enhancing mitochondrial function and reducing oxidative stress, allowing the brain to perform optimally.

How Methylene Blue Improves Depression and Anxiety

1. **Boosts Mitochondrial Energy Production:** Methylene blue acts as an electron donor in the brain's mitochondria, "jump-starting" energy production in cells that are underperforming. This means more ATP is generated, helping brain cells function better.
   - **Impact:** Increased energy improves cognitive function, mood stability, and emotional resilience.

2. **Reduces Oxidative Stress:** Oxidative stress leads to inflammation and damage in brain cells, which can worsen symptoms of depression and anxiety. Methylene blue acts as a potent antioxidant, neutralizing free radicals and reducing inflammation.
   - **Impact:** Protecting neurons leads to improved brain health and clearer thinking.

3. **Regulates Neurotransmitters:** Methylene blue has been shown to modulate the activity of key neurotransmitters, including serotonin and dopamine. These chemicals play a critical role in mood regulation.
   - **Impact:** Balanced serotonin and dopamine levels result in improved mood, reduced anxiety, and a greater sense of calm.

Methylene Blue and PTSD

PTSD is often linked to traumatic memories that are emotionally intense and difficult to process. Methylene blue is being explored for its ability to reduce the emotional charge of these memories during therapy.

- During trauma-focused therapy, methylene blue may help enhance memory reconsolidation, a process where memories are updated and re-stored.
- By improving energy and neurotransmitter balance, methylene blue can make the brain more receptive to therapeutic processes, allowing patients to process trauma more effectively.

Emerging Research: Early studies show that methylene blue, when combined with therapy, reduces PTSD symptoms by decreasing the emotional impact of traumatic memories.

Real-World Benefits and Emerging Evidence

As research into methylene blue expands, its potential to address challenging health conditions becomes clearer. Real-world results, combined with emerging scientific evidence, highlight its transformative benefits for mental health, skin rejuvenation, and even chronic illnesses. Here's a step-by-step look at how methylene blue is making waves in cutting-edge applications and delivering tangible results.

1. **Mental Health:** Depression, Anxiety, and PTSD: Clinical studies have shown methylene blue's profound effects on mood disorders. Its ability to optimize mitochondrial function, reduce oxidative stress, and modulate serotonin pathways makes it a unique approach to improving mental health.
   - In a double-blind study, low doses of methylene blue were found to reduce symptoms of depression and anxiety more effectively than a placebo. Participants reported better energy levels, improved emotional stability, and greater mental clarity.

- In PTSD therapy, methylene blue is emerging as an adjunct tool. When paired with trauma-focused therapy, it helps reduce the emotional intensity of traumatic memories, making healing faster and more effective.

2. **Skin Health and Anti-Aging:** Methylene blue's ability to protect cells from oxidative damage and boost collagen production makes it an exciting addition to anti-aging and skin health therapies.
   - In dermatological studies, topical methylene blue creams were shown to reduce fine lines, improve hydration, and enhance skin elasticity—results comparable to retinol but without irritation.
   - Methylene blue stimulates cellular repair and reduces inflammation, making it useful for wound healing, scar reduction, and improving conditions like rosacea.

3. **Chronic Conditions and Cancer Support:** Early research is exploring methylene blue's role in chronic conditions, including cancer, neurodegenerative diseases, and chronic fatigue syndrome.
   - **Cancer Support:** Methylene blue enhances oxygen utilization in cells, which can make cancer therapies like photodynamic therapy (PDT) more effective. Its role in reducing oxidative stress also helps support the immune system.
   - **Neurodegenerative Diseases:** Methylene blue slows the progression of Alzheimer's and Parkinson's by reducing protein misfolding and protecting neurons from damage.
   - **Chronic Fatigue:** By restoring mitochondrial function and energy production, methylene blue offers relief for those suffering from fatigue-related illnesses.

A Safe and Promising Approach

One of the most significant advantages of methylene blue is its safety profile when used correctly. Unlike many pharmaceutical treatments, it offers broad benefits with minimal side effects.

1. **Low Doses, Big Benefits:** Methylene blue is effective at low doses, often between *0.5–2 mg/kg of body weight* per day. This makes it a gentle yet powerful tool for health optimization and therapeutic use.
   - **For mental health:** Low doses are sufficient to boost mood, energy, and cognitive function.
   - **For skin health:** Topical formulations deliver benefits directly to the skin with little to no systemic side effects.

2. **Minimal Side Effects:** When used within safe guidelines, side effects are mild and manageable. The most common include temporary blue discoloration of urine and stool, which is completely harmless.
   - Nausea or dizziness can occur at higher doses but can be avoided by starting low and increasing gradually.

3. **A Complement to Existing Therapies:** Methylene blue does not replace existing treatments but can enhance and complement them. For instance:
   - It can work alongside therapy for PTSD or depression to improve outcomes.
   - As part of skin care, it adds a protective and rejuvenating layer to anti-aging protocols.
   - In cancer care, it may support photodynamic therapy and immune function.

SKIN HEALTH AND ANTI-AGING TREATMENTS

Aging is a natural process, but its visible signs—wrinkles, fine lines, and loss of elasticity—are often accelerated by environmental stress, oxidative damage, and declining cellular repair. Methylene blue has emerged as a cutting-edge solution in the world of skin health and anti-aging, offering a unique way to slow down and even reverse signs of aging. By targeting the underlying causes of skin decline at the cellular level, methylene blue stands out as a powerful and versatile tool for maintaining youthful, resilient skin.

How Methylene Blue Works at the Cellular Level

To understand how methylene blue delivers its powerful health and anti-aging effects, we need to look at its action at the cellular level. Aging and many health conditions are rooted in cellular decline, caused by mitochondrial dysfunction, oxidative stress, and inflammation. Methylene blue works by targeting these underlying causes, helping cells perform better, repair themselves, and remain resilient.

1. **Supporting Mitochondrial Function:** Mitochondria, the tiny power plants inside your cells, are responsible for producing energy in the form of ATP (adenosine triphosphate). As we age or experience stress, mitochondrial function declines, leading to fatigue, slower cellular repair, and visible signs of aging like wrinkles and sagging skin.
    *   **Methylene blue's role:** Methylene blue acts as an electron donor in the electron transport chain, a process that occurs in your mitochondria to create energy. When this process slows or stalls, methylene blue steps in to bridge the gaps, keeping the chain running smoothly and ensuring that cells continue to produce energy efficiently.
    *   **Why it matters:** By boosting ATP production, methylene blue improves cellular energy levels, which helps skin cells regenerate faster, maintain structure, and repair damage.

2. **Reducing Oxidative Stress:** Oxidative stress occurs when unstable molecules called free radicals build up in the body. These free radicals damage cells, proteins, and DNA, accelerating aging and contributing to diseases.
    *   **Methylene blue's role:** Methylene blue acts as a potent antioxidant, neutralizing free radicals and reducing oxidative stress. It protects cells from damage and inflammation, which are major drivers of aging and degenerative conditions.
    *   **Why it matters:** By shielding cells from oxidative stress, methylene blue prevents premature aging, supports healthier skin, and maintains overall cellular health.

3. **Enhancing Cellular Repair:** With better energy production and less oxidative stress, cells can focus on repairing and maintaining themselves. This includes producing collagen and elastin, the proteins responsible for firm, youthful skin. Methylene blue essentially gives your cells the tools they need to function optimally, combat aging, and stay resilient against environmental stressors.

Anti-Aging Benefits of Methylene Blue

By working at the cellular level, methylene blue offers a range of anti-aging benefits that improve skin health, repair damage, and slow visible signs of aging.

Here's how:

1. **Reduces Fine Lines and Wrinkles:** One of the primary benefits of methylene blue is its ability to stimulate the production of collagen and elastin, two proteins critical for skin elasticity and firmness. As mitochondrial energy improves, cells regenerate faster, leading to smoother, more youthful skin.
   - **Real-world impact:** Regular use of topical methylene blue has been shown to reduce the appearance of fine lines and improve overall skin texture without the irritation caused by other anti-aging treatments like retinoids.
2. **Improves Skin Hydration and Barrier Function:** Methylene blue helps repair the skin barrier, which is essential for retaining moisture and protecting against external stressors. By boosting cellular repair, methylene blue ensures your skin stays hydrated, plump, and healthy.
   - **Why this matters:** A stronger skin barrier keeps out pollutants and UV damage, two major contributors to premature aging.
3. **Protects Against UV and Environmental Damage:** Exposure to UV radiation and environmental toxins accelerates oxidative stress, leading to pigmentation, wrinkles, and dullness. Methylene blue's antioxidant properties neutralize free radicals, protecting skin cells from damage and reducing inflammation.
   - **How it helps:** This protection slows down the aging process and prevents the breakdown of skin structures.
4. **Speeds Up Wound Healing and Skin Regeneration:** Methylene blue promotes faster cellular turnover, which accelerates wound healing and reduces scars. Whether it's a cut, burn, or acne mark, methylene blue helps your skin regenerate efficiently and evenly.

How to Use Methylene Blue for Skin Health

Methylene blue is a breakthrough ingredient that's redefining skin care. It doesn't just mask the signs of aging—it works deep within your skin cells to repair damage, boost collagen, and fight the root causes of wrinkles and dullness. The best part? Using methylene blue for healthier, younger-looking skin is easier than you might think. In this section, you'll learn exactly how to incorporate it into your routine, step by step, and discover the impressive results it can deliver for anti-aging and overall skin health.

1. **Choose the Right Formulation:** To use methylene blue topically, it is essential to find high-quality formulations specifically designed for skin care. These may include:
   - **Serums:** Lightweight and easy to absorb, serums allow methylene blue to penetrate the skin effectively.
   - **Creams or Moisturizers:** These combine methylene blue with other nourishing ingredients to hydrate and repair the skin.
   - **Face Masks:** Methylene blue-infused masks provide deep hydration and rejuvenation during short treatment sessions.

Look for products that contain low concentrations of methylene blue (0.1–0.5%)—enough to deliver results without irritation.

2. **Cleanse and Prepare the Skin:** Start with a clean, dry face. Remove any dirt, oil, or makeup using a gentle cleanser. Properly prepped skin ensures that methylene blue can penetrate deeply and work more effectively.

3. **Apply Topically and Gently Massage**
   - Use a small amount of methylene blue serum or cream. A little goes a long way.
   - Apply the product evenly across your face, neck, or any areas of concern (e.g., fine lines, wrinkles, or dry patches).
   - Gently massage the product into the skin using upward, circular motions to stimulate blood flow and improve absorption.

4. **Combine with Other Skin Care Tools:** Methylene blue works synergistically with other proven biohacks:
   - Red Light Therapy: Applying methylene blue 10–15 minutes before a red light therapy session amplifies its benefits, enhancing cellular repair and energy production.
   - Hyaluronic Acid: Pairing methylene blue with hyaluronic acid locks in moisture, boosting hydration for plumper, smoother skin.
   - Vitamin C: This antioxidant duo can further protect the skin from oxidative damage and reduce pigmentation.

5. **Protect and Maintain Results**
   - Always apply sunscreen during the day. Methylene blue helps repair the skin, but UV exposure can still cause damage.
   - Use methylene blue products consistently—once or twice a day—for noticeable improvements over time.

Real-World Results and Emerging Evidence

The effectiveness of methylene blue for skin health is no longer just theoretical. Both clinical studies and real-world experiences highlight its remarkable ability to reduce signs of aging, improve skin texture, and promote cellular repair.

1. **Clinical Studies and Science-Backed Results:** Recent studies have shown that methylene blue is superior to traditional antioxidants like vitamin C and retinol in combating oxidative stress and supporting skin rejuvenation.
   - Improved Elasticity and Firmness: Research shows that methylene blue stimulates collagen and elastin production, resulting in firmer, plumper skin.
   - Reduced Fine Lines and Wrinkles: In a study comparing methylene blue with other anti-aging treatments, participants reported smoother skin and a visible reduction in fine lines after consistent use.
   - Enhanced Hydration: Methylene blue strengthens the skin barrier, helping it retain moisture for longer periods, which reduces dryness and flakiness.

2. **Real-World Experiences:** Countless individuals are turning to methylene blue as a game-changing solution for skin health. Here are some notable real-world outcomes:

   - Users report noticeable reductions in wrinkles and age spots after just a few weeks of using methylene blue serums.
   - Those with sensitive skin find methylene blue gentler than retinol, delivering similar anti-aging results without irritation.
   - People struggling with conditions like rosacea and eczema have shared improvements in skin texture, inflammation, and redness.

Case Example: A participant in an anti-aging trial experienced a 20% improvement in skin hydration and elasticity after applying a methylene blue cream daily for six weeks. Fine lines around the eyes and mouth were visibly diminished.

3. **A Future of Innovation:** As research continues, methylene blue is likely to play an even bigger role in dermatology and skin care. Its ability to repair skin at the cellular level and protect against aging is opening doors to innovative treatments for:

   - Chronic Skin Conditions: Like acne scars, rosacea, and hyperpigmentation.
   - Wound Healing: Accelerating the repair of damaged or injured skin.
   - Preventative Skin Care: Keeping skin healthier and more resilient as we age.

A New Era for Skin Health

Methylene blue offers a promising, science-backed approach to skin health and anti-aging. By targeting the root causes of skin damage—oxidative stress and mitochondrial decline—it rejuvenates your skin from the inside out. Whether you're looking to reduce wrinkles, improve hydration, or heal damaged skin, methylene blue is a versatile, forward-thinking solution that continues to reveal its potential. With consistent use and emerging research, it's clear that methylene blue isn't just another trend—it's a revolutionary step forward in skin care and wellness.

A Forward-Thinking Solution for Skin Health

Methylene blue is a game-changer in the fight against skin aging and damage. By addressing the root causes of cellular decline—oxidative stress and mitochondrial dysfunction—it offers a smarter, more effective way to maintain youthful, vibrant skin. Whether used for anti-aging, wound healing, or protecting against environmental stress, methylene blue is opening new possibilities for skin health and longevity. As research continues to expand, its role in dermatology and skin care is only just beginning to shine.

EXPLORING ITS POTENTIAL IN CANCER AND CHRONIC CONDITIONS

Methylene blue is proving to be more than just a health-boosting supplement—it's emerging as a potential ally in some of the toughest battles in modern medicine. From supporting cancer therapies to managing chronic conditions like neurodegenerative diseases and chronic fatigue, its ability to improve cellular function and reduce oxidative stress is showing exciting promise. While research is ongoing, the possibilities are inspiring. This section explores how methylene blue may complement existing treatments and offer new hope to those dealing with complex health challenges.

Methylene Blue and Cancer Support

Cancer is one of the most challenging health conditions to treat, often requiring a combination of therapies to target abnormal cell growth. Methylene blue, while not a cure, has shown promise as a supportive tool in cancer care. Its unique properties—enhancing cellular oxygen utilization, reducing oxidative stress, and disrupting cancer cell metabolism—position it as a valuable complement to conventional cancer treatments.

1. **Enhancing Photodynamic Therapy (PDT):** Photodynamic therapy is a treatment that uses light-sensitive compounds and specific wavelengths of light to generate reactive oxygen species (ROS), which selectively destroy cancer cells. Methylene blue is an effective photosensitizer, meaning it becomes activated when exposed to light, amplifying the effects of PDT.
   - **How it works:** Methylene blue accumulates in cancerous cells. When exposed to light, it produces ROS that damage and kill the cancer cells while sparing healthy ones.
   - **Benefits:** By increasing the precision of PDT, methylene blue reduces the side effects typically associated with broader cancer treatments.

2. **Targeting Mitochondrial Dysfunction in Cancer Cells:** Cancer cells often rely on abnormal mitochondrial function to fuel their rapid growth. Methylene blue interferes with this process.
   - **How it helps:**
     - Methylene blue disrupts the altered energy production in cancer cells, making it harder for them to survive and proliferate.
     - It enhances oxygen availability in healthy cells, supporting overall cellular health and helping the immune system target cancer more effectively.

3. **Protecting Healthy Cells During Treatment:** Traditional cancer treatments like chemotherapy and radiation can damage healthy cells. Methylene blue's antioxidant properties help protect these cells by reducing oxidative stress and promoting repair.
   - **Emerging Evidence:** Early studies indicate that methylene blue, when used in combination with chemotherapy or radiation, may enhance treatment efficacy while mitigating side effects like fatigue and tissue damage.

Managing Chronic Conditions

Chronic conditions such as neurodegenerative diseases, chronic fatigue syndrome (CFS), and autoimmune disorders often stem from underlying issues like mitochondrial dysfunction, inflammation, and oxidative stress. Methylene blue's ability to address these root causes makes it a promising therapeutic tool for managing these complex conditions.

1. **Neurodegenerative Diseases:** Diseases like Alzheimer's and Parkinson's involve the build-up of misfolded proteins and oxidative damage in the brain.

- **How methylene blue helps:**
  - It reduces protein misfolding and prevents the clumping of tau proteins, a hallmark of Alzheimer's disease.
  - By boosting mitochondrial function, it improves brain energy levels, supporting cognitive performance and slowing neurodegeneration.
- **Hopeful Impact:** Methylene blue's neuroprotective effects offer a new avenue for managing symptoms and improving quality of life for individuals with neurodegenerative diseases.

2. **Chronic Fatigue Syndrome and Fibromyalgia:** These conditions are often linked to systemic mitochondrial dysfunction and chronic inflammation, leading to severe fatigue and muscle pain.
   - **How methylene blue helps:**
     - Enhances mitochondrial energy production, reducing fatigue and improving stamina.
     - Acts as an anti-inflammatory agent, helping to alleviate pain and promote recovery.

3. **Autoimmune and Inflammatory Disorders:** In autoimmune conditions like rheumatoid arthritis or lupus, the immune system attacks healthy tissue, leading to chronic inflammation and damage.
   - **How methylene blue helps:**
     - Regulates overactive immune responses, reducing inflammation and protecting tissues from damage.
     - Supports cellular repair, helping to restore normal function in affected areas.
   - **Emerging Research:** Studies suggest that methylene blue's anti-inflammatory and antioxidant effects may play a role in slowing disease progression and improving symptoms in autoimmune disorders.

A New Frontier in Wellness

Methylene blue's ability to support cancer therapies and manage chronic conditions highlights its versatility as a therapeutic tool. By targeting mitochondrial dysfunction and oxidative stress—two common factors in many diseases—it addresses the root causes of complex health challenges.

While more research is needed, early findings are hopeful. Methylene blue offers a safe, complementary approach that can enhance traditional treatments and provide relief for individuals seeking innovative solutions for chronic and life-threatening conditions. Its expanding role in health care signals a promising future, inspiring hope for better management and improved outcomes.

Safety and Complementary Use

Methylene blue is not a standalone cure for cancer or chronic conditions but serves as a complementary tool to enhance existing therapies.

- **Low Doses, High Impact:** Methylene blue is effective at low doses, reducing the risk of side effects when used correctly.
- **Pairing with Conventional Treatments:** When combined with standard treatments like chemotherapy or mitochondrial supplements, methylene blue can amplify results without adding significant toxicity.

Hope for the Future

The potential applications of methylene blue in cancer and chronic conditions are vast, with ongoing research continuing to uncover its benefits. For individuals seeking innovative ways to support their health, methylene blue offers a safe, science-backed option that works by addressing the cellular root causes of disease.

As we look forward, methylene blue represents a beacon of hope in the fight against cancer and the management of chronic illnesses. Its unique ability to enhance cellular health and complement modern therapies makes it an exciting frontier in wellness and medical science.

CHAPTER 7: METHYLENE BLUE FOR EVERYDAY WELLNESS

Methylene blue isn't just for fixing problems—it's a tool you can use every day to stay ahead of them. Whether it's keeping your energy steady, staying sharp under pressure, or building resilience against stress, methylene blue can help you feel and perform your best. In this chapter, you'll learn how to incorporate methylene blue into your daily routine, practical ways to use it effectively for long-term health, and real stories of people who've used it to transform their lives. Let's explore how methylene blue can become a simple yet powerful part of your wellness journey.

BUILDING RESILIENCE WITH METHYLENE BLUE

Resilience is your body's ability to adapt to stress, recover from challenges, and maintain balance in the face of life's demands. Whether it's physical fatigue, mental pressure, or environmental stressors, resilience keeps you strong and stable. Methylene blue is a powerful tool for enhancing resilience because it works at the cellular level to optimize energy production, reduce oxidative stress, and support overall wellness. By incorporating methylene blue into your daily routine, you can build a foundation of strength and adaptability. Here's how to do it, step by step.

Understand How Methylene Blue Builds Resilience

1. **Cellular Energy Production:** Resilience starts in the mitochondria, the energy powerhouses of your cells. Methylene blue enhances mitochondrial function by acting as an electron donor, which ensures the efficient production of ATP (adenosine triphosphate). This boost in cellular energy improves your ability to recover from physical exertion, mental strain, and immune challenges.
   - **Benefits:** Increased stamina, quicker recovery, and sustained energy throughout the day.

2. **Fighting Oxidative Stress:** Everyday factors like pollution, stress, and poor diet generate free radicals that damage cells and tissues. Over time, this oxidative stress can weaken resilience and lead to fatigue, inflammation, and chronic issues. Methylene blue is a potent antioxidant that neutralizes free radicals and prevents cellular damage.
   - **Benefits:** Reduced inflammation, stronger immunity, and protection against aging.

3. **Enhancing Brain and Emotional Resilience:** Stress and mental pressure can leave you feeling drained and unfocused. Methylene blue supports brain health by improving neurotransmitter balance and increasing blood flow to key areas. It helps you stay calm, focused, and adaptable, even during high-pressure situations.
   - **Benefits:** Better mood stability, sharper focus, and improved decision-making under stress.

Incorporate Methylene Blue into Your Routine

1. **Establish Consistency:** Resilience is built over time, so regular use of methylene blue is key. Start with a low daily dose (0.5–1 mg/kg body weight) and gradually adjust based on how your body responds. Take it in the morning or during periods of high demand for the best results.

2. **Pair Methylene Blue with Lifestyle Habits:** Methylene blue works best when combined with a holistic approach to health. Here are some practices to amplify its effects:
   - Healthy Diet: Include antioxidant-rich foods like leafy greens, berries, and healthy fats to complement methylene blue's oxidative stress-reducing properties.
   - Stress Management: Practices like meditation, yoga, or breathing exercises enhance methylene blue's impact on emotional and cognitive resilience.
   - Exercise: Physical activity boosts mitochondrial health, and methylene blue can improve endurance and recovery.

3. **Stay Hydrated:** Proper hydration supports methylene blue's role in energy production and detoxification. Drink plenty of water throughout the day to maximize its benefits.

Real-Life Success Stories

Hearing how others have successfully incorporated methylene blue into their daily routines can inspire and motivate you to take action in your own wellness journey. From busy professionals to active seniors, methylene blue has become a cornerstone for many individuals looking to boost energy, improve focus, and build resilience. Here are three real-life success stories that showcase the transformative potential of this remarkable compound.

Case 1: The Corporate Professional Seeking Mental Clarity

- **Background:** Emma, a 39-year-old marketing executive, often struggled with brain fog and afternoon energy crashes. Her demanding job required sharp focus and creativity, but she found it increasingly difficult to maintain her productivity throughout the day.

Methylene Blue Integration:
   - Emma started taking *0.5 mg/kg* of methylene blue daily in the morning. She combined this with a high-protein breakfast and 10 minutes of mindfulness meditation to start her day with focus.
   - To complement methylene blue's effects, she added red light therapy to her evening routine, helping her unwind and enhance mitochondrial repair.

- **Results:** Within two weeks, Emma noticed significant improvements in her ability to concentrate during long meetings. Her energy levels remained steady throughout the day, and she felt more creative during brainstorming sessions. "It's like a fog has lifted," she said. "I can stay sharp and productive without the need for caffeine or sugary snacks."

Case 2: The Active Parent Finding Balance

- **Background:** Michael, a 42-year-old father of two, found himself drained by the dual demands of parenting and maintaining an active lifestyle. Between work, family commitments, and his passion for weekend cycling, Michael struggled with fatigue and slow recovery after workouts.

<u>Methylene Blue Integration:</u>
- Michael began using methylene blue sublingually before his morning workouts at a dose of ***1 mg/kg***
- He also focused on staying hydrated and consuming antioxidant-rich foods, such as berries and leafy greens, to complement methylene blue's benefits.

- **Results:** Michael quickly noticed an improvement in his endurance during cycling sessions and a faster recovery time afterward. His newfound energy also allowed him to engage more fully with his kids. "It's like I've regained my edge. I can push myself physically and still have the energy to play soccer with my kids in the evening."

Case 3: The Senior Embracing Healthy Aging
- **Background:** Linda, a 68-year-old retiree, wanted to maintain her independence and vitality as she aged. She had minor concerns about memory lapses and joint stiffness, which she hoped to address with a holistic wellness approach.

<u>Methylene Blue Integration:</u>
- Linda started with a low dose of ***0.5 mg/kg*** methylene blue, taken daily after breakfast.
- She paired methylene blue with a regular yoga practice and a diet rich in omega-3 fatty acids to support brain health and mobility.
- To track her progress, Linda kept a wellness journal, noting changes in her energy, mood, and memory.

- **Results:** Over several months, Linda experienced improved mental clarity and a reduction in joint discomfort. She also felt more engaged in her hobbies, such as gardening and painting. "I feel sharper and more active than I have in years. Methylene blue has become my secret weapon for staying young at heart."

Takeaway Lessons
These success stories highlight the versatility of methylene blue in meeting diverse wellness goals.

<u>Here's what we can learn:</u>

1. **Consistency Is Key:** Each individual achieved results by using methylene blue regularly and combining it with healthy habits.

2. **Pairing with Lifestyle Choices Amplifies Benefits:** Whether it's mindfulness, exercise, or a nutritious diet, methylene blue works best when part of a comprehensive routine.

3. **Tracking Progress Enhances Success:** Keeping a journal or monitoring changes with wearable devices can help you stay motivated and adjust your protocol as needed.

PRACTICAL TIPS FOR LONG-TERM USE

Incorporating methylene blue into your daily routine for long-term use can yield sustained benefits for energy, focus, and overall wellness. While the compound itself is effective, its true potential lies in how consistently and wisely you use it as part of a holistic lifestyle. The key is to develop habits that amplify its effects and support your body's resilience. Below is a step-by-step guide with practical tips to help you make methylene blue a seamless and sustainable part of your wellness routine.

Establish a Consistent Routine

- **Start Small and Build Gradually:** Consistency is critical to experiencing methylene blue's long-term benefits. Begin with a low daily dose, such as *0.5–1 mg per kilogram of body weight*, and adjust based on how your body responds.
    1. **Morning Routine:** Taking methylene blue in the morning can set a positive tone for the day, supporting energy and focus.
    2. **Before Demanding Tasks:** Use it before mentally or physically challenging activities for an added boost.

Stick to a Schedule: For best results, take methylene blue at the same time each day. This builds a habit and ensures a steady supply in your system to support cellular health and energy production.

Pair Methylene Blue with Healthy Habits

Methylene blue works best when integrated into a comprehensive approach to wellness. Here are some ways to complement its effects:

- **Support with Nutrition:** A nutrient-rich diet enhances methylene blue's benefits. Focus on:
    1. **Antioxidant-Rich Foods:** Berries, leafy greens, and nuts to complement its role in reducing oxidative stress.
    2. **Healthy Fats:** Avocado, olive oil, and fatty fish to support mitochondrial function.
    3. **Hydration:** Drink plenty of water to aid cellular processes and enhance detoxification.

- **Combine with Stress Management Practices:** Chronic stress can weaken resilience and counteract progress. Pair methylene blue with stress-reducing practices:
    - **Meditation or Mindfulness:** These practices amplify methylene blue's positive effects on focus and emotional balance.
    - **Yoga or Gentle Exercise:** Improves blood flow and supports mitochondrial health, aligning with methylene blue's functions.

- **Incorporate Physical Activity:** Regular movement enhances methylene blue's ability to improve energy and recovery. Try:
    1. Cardio Workouts: Boosts oxygen flow and complements methylene blue's cellular oxygen utilization.
    2. Strength Training: Enhances muscle recovery when paired with methylene blue.

CHAPTER 8: FUTURE PERSPECTIVES ON METHYLENE BLUE

Methylene blue is on the verge of transforming health and wellness in ways we're only beginning to understand. Its current benefits are impressive, but what lies ahead is even more exciting. Scientists are uncovering new uses for methylene blue that could change how we think about aging, chronic diseases, and overall health optimization. In this chapter, we'll explore the cutting-edge research, its growing role in longevity science, and innovative technologies that promise to make methylene blue even more powerful and accessible. The future is bright, and methylene blue is leading the way.

EMERGING RESEARCH AND BREAKTHROUGHS

Methylene blue is more than a tried-and-true compound—it's becoming a key player in cutting-edge health research. Scientists are uncovering its potential to address chronic diseases, support healthy aging, and even enhance daily performance. As new studies reveal its impact on cellular health and innovative delivery methods make it easier to use, methylene blue is emerging as a powerful tool for the future of health and wellness. This section dives into the latest breakthroughs and shows how methylene blue is poised to change the way we think about prevention, longevity, and optimization.

Advancements in Brain Health and Neuroprotection

Methylene blue has long been recognized for its ability to enhance mitochondrial function and reduce oxidative stress, making it a promising candidate for addressing neurodegenerative diseases.

1. **Alzheimer's and Parkinson's Diseases:** Recent studies are investigating methylene blue's ability to prevent tau protein aggregation, a hallmark of Alzheimer's disease, and protect neurons from oxidative damage linked to Parkinson's.
   - **Breakthrough Insight:** A clinical trial showed that low doses of methylene blue could slow cognitive decline in early-stage Alzheimer's patients.
2. **Traumatic Brain Injury (TBI):** Research is exploring methylene blue's ability to stabilize mitochondrial function and improve recovery outcomes in individuals with TBI.
3. **Cognitive Performance in Healthy Individuals:** Beyond disease management, early studies suggest methylene blue could enhance focus, memory, and decision-making in healthy adults by boosting brain energy metabolism.

Expanding Applications in Chronic Disease Management

Chronic conditions like diabetes, cardiovascular disease, and autoimmune disorders often stem from mitochondrial dysfunction, oxidative stress, and systemic inflammation—areas where methylene blue excels.

- **Diabetes:** Methylene blue has shown promise in improving insulin sensitivity by reducing inflammation and oxidative stress in pancreatic cells. This could potentially slow the progression of type 2 diabetes.
- **Cardiovascular Health:** By improving oxygen utilization and mitochondrial function, methylene blue is being studied for its role in enhancing cardiac efficiency, potentially benefiting individuals with heart failure or ischemic conditions.
- **Autoimmune Diseases:** Researchers are exploring methylene blue's potential to regulate overactive immune responses, offering hope for conditions like rheumatoid arthritis or lupus.

Longevity Science and Aging Research

Longevity science focuses on extending not just lifespan but also healthspan—the number of years lived in good health. Methylene blue's impact on cellular health positions it as a key player in this field.

- **Mitochondrial Health and Cellular Aging:** Studies have shown that methylene blue helps maintain mitochondrial function and protects against the oxidative damage that accelerates aging.
- **Breakthrough Insight:** By reducing DNA damage and supporting telomere integrity, methylene blue is being explored as a potential anti-aging therapy.
- **Autophagy Activation:** Early research indicates methylene blue may enhance autophagy, the body's natural process of clearing out damaged cells, promoting healthier tissues and slowing age-related decline.

Innovations in Delivery Systems

As research into methylene blue continues, scientists are developing innovative delivery systems to enhance its effectiveness, convenience, and precision. These advancements aim to maximize methylene blue's therapeutic potential while minimizing side effects, making it more accessible for a wide range of applications. Let's explore the cutting-edge methods shaping the future of methylene blue use.

1. **Nanoformulations for Targeted Delivery:** Nanoformulations involve encapsulating methylene blue in nanoparticles, which allows for precise targeting of specific tissues or organs. This technology significantly improves its bioavailability, meaning more of the compound reaches the intended site of action.
   - **How It Works:** Nanoparticles can carry methylene blue directly to areas of need, such as the brain, muscles, or mitochondria. This reduces waste and enhances efficacy.
   - **Benefits:**
     - Higher absorption rates and faster results.
     - Reduced side effects by limiting exposure to unintended areas.
     - Enhanced effectiveness in treating localized conditions, such as neurodegenerative diseases or certain types of cancer.

2. **Transdermal Patches for Steady Absorption:** Transdermal patches are an exciting innovation for delivering methylene blue through the skin. These patches release small, consistent doses over time, providing a steady supply without the need for frequent dosing.
   - **How It Works:** The patch is applied to the skin, allowing methylene blue to enter the bloodstream gradually.
   - **Benefits:**
     - Convenient for daily use without the need for measuring doses.
     - Ideal for individuals seeking long-term, low-dose benefits.
     - Reduces peaks and troughs in effectiveness, offering more stable results.

3. **Intranasal Delivery for Brain Health:** Intranasal sprays are being developed to deliver methylene blue directly to the brain through the nasal passages. This method bypasses the digestive system and blood-brain barrier, ensuring rapid effects on cognitive function.
   - **How It Works:** The spray is administered into the nostrils, where it is absorbed through the nasal mucosa and transported directly to the brain.
   - **Benefits:**
     - Quick and targeted effects for enhancing focus, memory, and mental clarity.
     - Promising for managing neurodegenerative diseases or acute cognitive challenges.

4. **Combination Therapies and Stacking Innovations:** Researchers are also exploring how methylene blue can be combined with other compounds, such as NAD+ precursors or antioxidants, for synergistic benefits. These combinations may amplify its effects on energy, recovery, and aging.

Staying Informed and Embracing the Future

The field of methylene blue research is rapidly evolving, and staying informed is key to leveraging its full potential. As new discoveries and technologies emerge, being proactive about education and experimentation can help you make the most of this powerful compound.

1. **Follow the Latest Research:** Keep up with new studies and clinical trials to stay ahead of the curve. Subscribe to reputable medical journals, follow wellness experts, or join biohacking communities to learn about advancements in methylene blue applications.
2. **Experiment Safely and Wisely:** As new delivery systems and formulations become available, work with a healthcare provider to ensure you're using them effectively and safely. Start with small doses and track your results to identify what works best for your unique needs.
3. **Be Open to Emerging Uses:** The future of methylene blue is filled with possibilities. Scientists are exploring its applications in areas like cancer therapy, chronic disease management, and even space medicine for addressing cellular challenges in extreme environments. Embrace the potential for these innovations to improve your health and well-being.
4. **Share Your Experiences:** By documenting your journey with methylene blue, you can contribute to a growing body of knowledge. Sharing your results may inspire others to explore its benefits while promoting responsible and informed use.

A New Era for Methylene Blue

Methylene blue is at the forefront of groundbreaking health research, offering hope for those looking to enhance wellness, combat chronic diseases, and support longevity. With ongoing breakthroughs in its applications and delivery methods, its future as a cornerstone of health optimization is brighter than ever. As the science evolves, methylene blue continues to prove itself as a versatile and indispensable tool for the next generation of health solutions.

THE ROLE OF METHYLENE BLUE IN LONGEVITY SCIENCE

Longevity science focuses on living healthier, not just longer. It's about understanding aging at its core and finding ways to slow or even reverse its effects. Methylene blue is gaining attention as a powerful tool in this field, thanks to its ability to protect cells, boost energy, and fight oxidative damage. With exciting research highlighting its role in maintaining vitality and slowing cellular aging, methylene blue is shaping the future of health and wellness. Let's dive into how this remarkable compound is unlocking new possibilities for staying strong, sharp, and energized as we age.

Understanding Cellular Aging

Aging is a natural process driven by the gradual decline of cellular health. Two key factors contribute to this decline:

1. **Mitochondrial Dysfunction:** Mitochondria, the energy factories of our cells, produce ATP (adenosine triphosphate), which powers every process in the body. Over time, mitochondria become less efficient, leading to lower energy production and increased oxidative stress.
2. **Oxidative Damage and Inflammation:** Aging cells accumulate oxidative damage from free radicals, unstable molecules that damage DNA, proteins, and lipids. This damage accelerates aging and contributes to chronic diseases.

Methylene blue directly addresses these issues, making it a key player in longevity science.

How Methylene Blue Supports Longevity

1. **Enhancing Mitochondrial Function:** Methylene blue is a potent mitochondrial enhancer. By acting as an electron donor, it improves the efficiency of the electron transport chain, the process mitochondria use to produce ATP.
   - **Why It Matters:** Better mitochondrial function means more energy for cellular repair and regeneration, processes that decline with age.
   - **Impact:** Increased vitality, reduced fatigue, and healthier aging at the cellular level.

2. **Reducing Oxidative Stress:** Methylene blue is also a powerful antioxidant. It neutralizes free radicals and prevents oxidative damage, protecting cells from wear and tear.
   - **Why It Matters:** Reducing oxidative stress helps prevent age-related cellular damage, supporting longer-lasting health and vitality.

3.   **Supporting Cellular Repair Mechanisms:** Methylene blue stimulates autophagy, the body's process of clearing out damaged cells and recycling their components.
   - **Why It Matters:** Efficient cellular repair keeps tissues and organs functioning optimally, reducing the risk of age-related diseases.

Recent Breakthroughs in Longevity Research

Longevity research has made remarkable strides in recent years, and methylene blue is emerging as a key player in this groundbreaking field. Studies are uncovering its potential to address the fundamental drivers of aging and promote a longer, healthier life. Here's a closer look at the recent breakthroughs.

1.   **Protecting Mitochondrial Function:** Mitochondria, the energy centers of our cells, are crucial for health and longevity. As we age, mitochondrial efficiency declines, leading to fatigue, inflammation, and cellular damage. Methylene blue has demonstrated an ability to restore mitochondrial function by enhancing ATP production and reducing oxidative stress.
   - **Recent Findings:** A study revealed that methylene blue improves mitochondrial respiration, enabling cells to produce energy more efficiently. This effect is particularly significant in tissues with high energy demands, like the brain, heart, and muscles.
   - **Impact:** This breakthrough positions methylene blue as a potential therapy for age-related conditions like neurodegeneration and muscle weakness.

2.   **Reducing Oxidative Damage:** Oxidative stress, caused by an imbalance between free radicals and antioxidants, is a major contributor to aging. Methylene blue's antioxidant properties protect cells by neutralizing free radicals and preventing DNA damage.
   - **Recent Findings:** Research shows that methylene blue reduces oxidative stress markers in animal models of aging. In human studies, it has been linked to improved skin health and reduced signs of aging.
   - **Impact:** By minimizing oxidative damage, methylene blue helps preserve cellular integrity and function, delaying the onset of age-related diseases.

3.   **Preserving Telomere Length:** Telomeres, the protective caps at the ends of chromosomes, shorten as cells divide, contributing to aging. Emerging evidence suggests that methylene blue may help maintain telomere length by reducing cellular stress.
   - **Recent Findings:** Preliminary studies have shown that methylene blue enhances the activity of enzymes involved in telomere preservation, slowing cellular aging.
   - **Impact:** This breakthrough highlights methylene blue's potential in extending healthspan by supporting genomic stability.

Future Innovations in Longevity Science

The future of methylene blue in longevity science is filled with exciting possibilities. Researchers are exploring advanced delivery systems and synergistic therapies to maximize its effectiveness.

1.   **Nanoformulations for Precision Delivery:** Nanoformulations involve encapsulating methylene blue in tiny particles designed to deliver it directly to target cells or tissues.

- **Advancements:** These formulations enhance bioavailability, allowing for smaller doses with greater effectiveness. Targeted delivery could focus on specific areas, such as the brain or heart.
- **Potential:** Nanoformulations could revolutionize the use of methylene blue in treating age-related conditions by reducing side effects and optimizing results.

2. **Combination Therapies:** Combining methylene blue with other compounds, like NAD+ precursors or senolytics, could amplify its effects.
   - **Advancements:** Researchers are investigating how these combinations can enhance mitochondrial function, clear damaged cells, and boost cellular repair.
   - **Potential:** Such therapies could provide a comprehensive approach to addressing aging at multiple levels.

3. **Personalized Longevity Protocols:** As research advances, the future of methylene blue lies in personalized medicine. Genetic testing and biomarker analysis could help create tailored protocols that maximize its benefits for each individual.
   - **Advancements:** AI and data-driven health tools are making it easier to customize treatments.
   - **Potential:** Personalized protocols could optimize the timing, dosage, and combination of methylene blue with other interventions.

Staying Informed About Methylene Blue's Role in Longevity

Longevity science is evolving rapidly, and methylene blue is at the forefront. Here's how to stay engaged:

- **Follow the Research:** Stay updated on clinical trials and studies exploring methylene blue's potential in aging and age-related diseases.
- **Experiment with Guidance:** Work with a healthcare provider to incorporate methylene blue safely into your wellness routine.
- **Be Open to Innovation:** As new formulations and delivery methods become available, consider how they might fit into your longevity strategy.

INNOVATIONS AND FUTURE APPLICATIONS

Methylene blue is just beginning to show its full potential. While it's already recognized for boosting energy, enhancing focus, and supporting cellular health, ongoing research is uncovering ways to make it even more effective and accessible. With new delivery systems, cutting-edge technologies, and promising therapeutic combinations on the horizon, methylene blue is set to transform health and wellness in ways we couldn't have imagined. Let's explore the exciting innovations that are shaping its future and the groundbreaking possibilities ahead.

Nanoformulations for Enhanced Effectiveness

Nanoformulations are leading the charge in methylene blue innovation. By encapsulating the compound in nanoparticles, scientists can enhance its bioavailability and target it to specific tissues or cells.

How It Works:
- Nanoparticles act as delivery vehicles, carrying methylene blue directly to its intended destination, such as mitochondria, neurons, or cancer cells.
- This precise targeting reduces the amount of methylene blue required while amplifying its therapeutic effects.

Benefits:
- Improved absorption and effectiveness.
- Minimized side effects by avoiding unintended tissues.
- More focused applications for conditions like neurodegenerative diseases and localized infections.

Visionary Impact: Imagine methylene blue being used to treat specific areas of the brain affected by Alzheimer's or Parkinson's with unparalleled precision.

Transdermal and Time-Release Systems

Innovative delivery systems are making methylene blue more user-friendly and consistent in its effects.

Transdermal Patches: These patches deliver methylene blue through the skin, offering a steady release over time.
- **Advantages:** Convenient for daily use, eliminates the need for frequent dosing, and maintains stable blood levels throughout the day.
- **Potential Uses:** Ideal for individuals using methylene blue for energy, focus, or chronic conditions that require long-term treatment.

Time-Release Capsules: These advanced formulations gradually release methylene blue over a set period.
- **Advantages:** Prevents peaks and troughs in effectiveness, reduces the frequency of administration, and ensures consistent benefits.

Visionary Impact: These systems could simplify methylene blue use, making it more accessible to a broader population while enhancing compliance.

Intranasal Delivery for Brain Health

The potential of methylene blue for brain health is immense, and intranasal delivery systems are being developed to maximize its cognitive benefits.

How It Works:
- Intranasal sprays deliver methylene blue directly to the brain via the nasal passages, bypassing the blood-brain barrier.
- This method ensures rapid absorption and targeted action.

Benefits:
- Quick effects on focus, memory, and clarity.
- Potential for treating neurodegenerative diseases more efficiently.

Visionary Impact: Intranasal methylene blue could become a go-to option for professionals seeking sharper mental performance or patients managing cognitive decline.

Synergistic Therapies and Combinations

Researchers are exploring how methylene blue can be combined with other compounds to amplify its effects.

Combinations in Development:
- **With NAD+ Precursors:** For enhanced mitochondrial repair and energy production.
- **With Senolytics:** To clear damaged cells while methylene blue protects and restores healthy ones.
- **With Red Light Therapy:** Combining methylene blue with light activation for photodynamic treatments targeting infections or cancer.

Visionary Impact: These combinations could redefine therapies for chronic diseases, aging, and even athletic recovery.

Personalized Medicine and AI Integration

The future of methylene blue lies in its integration into personalized medicine, where treatments are tailored to the individual's genetic profile, health markers, and lifestyle.

How It Will Work:
- Advances in AI and wearable technology will analyze real-time data on an individual's health, recommending optimized methylene blue doses and delivery methods.
- Genetic testing could identify how a person metabolizes methylene blue, further personalizing its use.

Visionary Impact: Personalized methylene blue protocols could become a cornerstone of preventative and precision medicine, helping individuals achieve peak health and longevity.

CHAPTER 9: RESOURCES AND APPENDICES

This chapter serves as your go-to toolkit for all things methylene blue, designed to simplify your journey and empower you with practical resources. From understanding key terms to quick-reference guides and trusted product recommendations, you'll find everything you need to confidently incorporate methylene blue into your wellness routine.

GLOSSARY OF TERMS

The glossary provides clear and simple explanations of key terms related to methylene blue, helping you navigate the concepts discussed in this book. Whether you're revisiting scientific principles or learning new terminology, this glossary is your quick-reference guide.

- **Acidosis:** A condition where there is too much acid in the body's fluids; methylene blue helps maintain proper pH balance in cells.
- **Aerobic Respiration:** The process by which cells produce energy using oxygen, enhanced by methylene blue.
- **Anaerobic Respiration:** Energy production in the absence of oxygen; methylene blue helps cells optimize this process.
- **Antioxidant:** A molecule that neutralizes free radicals, preventing oxidative damage to cells.
- **Apoptosis:** Programmed cell death; methylene blue supports healthy apoptosis to remove damaged cells.
- **ATP (Adenosine Triphosphate):** The main energy currency of cells, produced by mitochondria to fuel cellular functions.
- **Autophagy:** The body's process of clearing out damaged cells, essential for anti-aging and cellular repair.
- **Bioavailability:** The proportion of a substance that enters the bloodstream and becomes available for use by the body.
- **Biohacking:** A lifestyle approach that uses science and technology to enhance health and performance; methylene blue is a key tool for many biohackers.
- **Biomarker:** A measurable indicator of health or disease; methylene blue's effects can improve key biomarkers like oxidative stress levels.
- **Blood-Brain Barrier:** A selective barrier that protects the brain by filtering substances in the bloodstream; methylene blue can cross this barrier.
- **Blue Urine:** A harmless side effect of methylene blue caused by its excretion through the urinary tract.
- **Cardioprotection:** The ability to protect the heart from damage; methylene blue offers cardioprotective effects.

- **Cellular Repair:** The process of restoring cell function and structure, facilitated by methylene blue.
- **Chronic Conditions:** Long-term health issues, such as diabetes or neurodegenerative diseases, that often involve mitochondrial dysfunction.
- **Chronic Fatigue Syndrome (CFS):** A condition characterized by extreme tiredness, often linked to mitochondrial dysfunction; methylene blue can help alleviate symptoms.
- **Cognitive Decline**: A reduction in mental abilities, often associated with aging; methylene blue supports brain health to counteract this.
- **Cognitive Function:** Mental processes like memory, attention, and problem-solving that methylene blue can enhance.
- **Cytoplasm:** The gel-like substance within cells where many metabolic processes occur.
- **Detoxification:** The process of removing toxins from the body; methylene blue aids in cellular detoxification.
- **DNA Damage:** Harm to the genetic material within cells, often caused by oxidative stress; methylene blue can help protect against this.
- **Dose Titration:** The process of adjusting a dose to find the most effective and safe level for an individual.
- **Dose-Response Relationship:** The correlation between the dose of a substance and its effects on the body.
- **Dual-Action Compound:** A substance with more than one therapeutic effect, such as methylene blue's roles as both an antioxidant and mitochondrial enhancer.
- **Electrophysiology:** The study of electrical activity in the body, particularly in cells; methylene blue can stabilize cellular electrical function.
- **Electron Donor:** A molecule that donates electrons in chemical reactions; methylene blue acts as one in the electron transport chain.
- **Electron Transport Chain:** A process in mitochondria that produces ATP; methylene blue helps improve its efficiency.
- **Endogenous Antioxidants:** Antioxidants naturally produced in the body; methylene blue complements their action.
- **Energy Metabolism:** The process of converting food and oxygen into energy; methylene blue enhances this at the cellular level.
- **Enzyme:** A protein that speeds up chemical reactions in the body, many of which are supported by methylene blue.
- **Epigenetics:** The study of how environmental factors affect gene expression; methylene blue may influence epigenetic markers of aging.
- **Free Radicals:** Unstable molecules that cause oxidative stress; neutralized by antioxidants like methylene blue.
- **Functional Medicine:** A medical approach focusing on root causes of disease; methylene blue aligns with this by addressing mitochondrial dysfunction.
- **Glutathione:** The body's master antioxidant, whose production is supported by methylene blue.
- **Hemoglobin:** A protein in red blood cells that carries oxygen; methylene blue can enhance its function in certain conditions.

- **Healthspan:** The number of years a person lives in good health, as opposed to total lifespan; a focus of longevity science.
- **Heavy Metals:** Toxic substances sometimes found in low-quality methylene blue products; avoid these impurities.
- **Hyperbaric Oxygen Therapy:** A treatment that delivers oxygen under pressure; sometimes combined with methylene blue for enhanced effects.
- **Immune Modulation:** Adjusting immune responses to achieve balance; methylene blue has immune-modulating properties.
- **Inflammation:** The body's response to injury or infection, which methylene blue can help reduce.
- **Intermittent Hypoxia:** Short periods of reduced oxygen, often used in biohacking; methylene blue supports recovery from hypoxic stress.
- **Intranasal Delivery:** A method of administering substances through the nasal passages, used for targeting the brain.
- **Ischemia:** Restricted blood flow to tissues; methylene blue can help protect cells during ischemic episodes.
- **Light-Activated Therapy:** A treatment where light activates a compound, such as methylene blue in photodynamic therapy.
- **Lipid Peroxidation:** The oxidative degradation of fats, damaging cell membranes; methylene blue reduces lipid peroxidation.
- **Longevity Science:** The study of extending healthy lifespan through biological and medical interventions.
- **Metabolic Health:** The state of optimal function of metabolic processes; methylene blue supports energy balance and efficiency.
- **Mitochondria:** Organelles in cells responsible for energy production; often referred to as the cell's "powerhouses."
- **Mitochondrial Dysfunction:** A decline in mitochondrial performance, linked to aging and chronic diseases.
- **Neurodegenerative Disease:** Conditions like Alzheimer's and Parkinson's that involve the gradual loss of brain function.
- **Neurogenesis:** The creation of new neurons; methylene blue is being studied for its potential to support this process.
- **Neurotransmitter:** Chemicals in the brain that transmit signals between nerve cells; methylene blue supports their balance.
- **Nitric Oxide:** A molecule that helps regulate blood flow and cellular signaling; methylene blue interacts with nitric oxide pathways to optimize function.
- **Nanoformulation:** A delivery method that uses nanoparticles to improve the precision and effectiveness of substances like methylene blue.
- **Oxidative Stress:** A harmful imbalance between free radicals and antioxidants in the body.
- **Photodynamic Therapy (PDT):** A treatment that uses light-activated compounds, such as methylene blue, to target specific cells.
- **Pro-oxidant:** A substance that can promote oxidation in high doses, opposite to an antioxidant.
- **Protein Aggregation:** The clumping of misfolded proteins, often linked to neurodegenerative diseases; methylene blue helps prevent this.

- **Reactive Oxygen Species (ROS):** Chemically reactive molecules that can damage cells; methylene blue reduces their impact.
- **Recovery:** The process of healing and restoring the body after stress or injury; methylene blue accelerates this.
- **Red Light Therapy:** A biohacking tool that uses red wavelengths of light to enhance mitochondrial function, often paired with methylene blue.
- **Resilience:** The body's ability to adapt to stress and recover from challenges, supported by methylene blue.
- **Senescence:** The process where cells stop dividing and accumulate damage, contributing to aging.
- **Senolytics:** Compounds that clear senescent cells, often paired with methylene blue for anti-aging benefits.
- **Sublingual Administration:** Taking a substance under the tongue for faster absorption into the bloodstream.
- **Systemic:** Relating to the entire body, as opposed to localized areas; methylene blue has systemic effects.
- **Telomeres:** Protective caps on the ends of chromosomes that shorten with age; methylene blue may help preserve their length.
- **Therapeutic Dose:** The amount of a substance required to achieve its desired health benefits.
- **Time-Release Capsule:** A delivery system that gradually releases methylene blue for sustained effects.
- **Topical Application:** Applying a substance to the skin, such as methylene blue for anti-aging benefits.
- **Toxicity:** The degree to which a substance can harm the body; methylene blue is safe when used correctly.
- **Transdermal Delivery:** Absorbing a substance through the skin, often via patches or creams.
- **Tumor Microenvironment:** The cellular environment around a tumor; methylene blue is being explored for targeted cancer therapies.
- **Ubiquinone (CoQ10):** A compound involved in mitochondrial energy production; methylene blue enhances similar pathways.
- **Wellness Optimization:** The proactive pursuit of peak physical and mental health using tools like methylene blue.
- **Xenobiotics:** Foreign substances in the body, such as pollutants; methylene blue can help mitigate their oxidative effects.
- **Youthful Aging:** Maintaining energy, clarity, and vitality throughout aging; a goal methylene blue supports.
- **Zinc Ionophore:** A substance that helps zinc enter cells, potentially boosting immunity; methylene blue shows similar mechanisms.
- **Zone of Inflammation:** Areas of the body affected by chronic inflammation, where methylene blue can provide relief.
- **Zygote:** The earliest stage of human development; mitochondrial health at this stage influences lifelong vitality.

QUICK REFERENCE DOSAGE AND BENEFITS GUIDE

To make your methylene blue journey as effective and straightforward as possible, this section provides a quick-reference guide to dosages and their associated benefits. Whether your goal is enhancing energy, improving cognition, or supporting longevity, understanding the right dosage and timing is essential. Use this as your go-to resource for incorporating methylene blue into your daily routine.

Understanding Dosage and Its Importance

When it comes to methylene blue, understanding dosage is crucial to unlocking its full potential safely and effectively. Because methylene blue's effects are dose-dependent, the right amount can make a significant difference, whether your goal is boosting energy, improving focus, or addressing specific health challenges. The key lies in finding the balance that suits your individual needs.

Why Dosage Matters:

- **Too Low:** A dose that is too small may not deliver noticeable benefits.
- **Too High:** Excessive doses can lead to side effects or diminish its effectiveness by acting as a pro-oxidant rather than an antioxidant.
- **Just Right:** A properly tailored dose ensures optimal results without unnecessary risks.

Methylene blue dosages are typically measured in **milligrams per kilogram (mg/kg)** of body weight, making it adaptable for users of all sizes. The ideal dosage depends on your health goals, the method of administration, and your body's unique response.

How to Start:

- **Begin Low:** Starting with a low dose allows you to observe how your body reacts.
- **Increase Gradually:** Adjust slowly as needed, tracking any improvements or side effects.
- **Stay Consistent:** Consistency in dosage and timing ensures stable benefits over time.

Dosage Recommendations Based on Goals

Different health and wellness objectives call for specific dosage ranges. Below are practical recommendations to help you align your methylene blue use with your personal goals.

1. **Boosting Energy and Reducing Fatigue**
    - **Dosage:** 0.5–1 mg/kg of body weight.
    - **Goal:** Enhance mitochondrial efficiency, increase ATP production, and provide a sustained energy boost.
    - **Timing:** Take in the morning or before energy-intensive activities to stay energized throughout the day.
    - **Example:** If you weigh 70 kg (154 lbs), start with 35–70 mg in the morning.

---

2. **Cognitive Enhancement**
   - **Dosage:** 0.5–1 mg/kg of body weight.
   - **Goal:** Improve focus, memory, and clarity by supporting brain energy metabolism and neurotransmitter balance.
   - **Timing:** Take 30–60 minutes before tasks that require intense mental effort, such as studying or problem-solving.
   - **Example:** For a 60 kg (132 lbs) individual, take 30–60 mg before starting a challenging work project.

3. **Anti-Aging and Longevity**
   - **Dosage:** 1–2 mg/kg of body weight.
   - **Goal:** Reduce oxidative stress, slow cellular aging, and promote autophagy for long-term health and vitality.
   - **Timing:** Take daily with a meal for sustained anti-aging benefits.
   - **Example:** A person weighing 80 kg (176 lbs) may take 80–160 mg once a day.

4. **Recovery from Stress or Exercise**
   - **Dosage:** 1–2 mg/kg of body weight.
   - **Goal:** Accelerate recovery by boosting cellular repair and reducing inflammation.
   - **Timing:** Take immediately after physical exertion or periods of high mental stress.
   - **Example:** A 65 kg (143 lbs) athlete could take 65–130 mg post-workout for faster recovery.

5. **Targeted Therapeutic Use**
   - **Dosage:** 2–3 mg/kg of body weight (under professional guidance).
   - **Goal:** Address chronic conditions like neurodegenerative diseases or mitochondrial disorders.
   - **Timing:** As prescribed by a healthcare provider, tailored to the specific condition.
   - **Example:** Under medical supervision, a 75 kg (165 lbs) individual might take 150–225 mg to support treatment goals.

Benefits Overview at a Glance

Methylene blue offers a wide range of benefits, making it a versatile tool for optimizing health and wellness. To help you quickly identify how methylene blue can support your specific goals, this section provides a concise benefits overview paired with recommended dosages and usage tips.

Goal	Dosage Range	Benefits	Timing
General Wellness	0.5–1 mg/kg	Boosts energy, reduces fatigue	Morning
Cognitive Enhancement	0.5–1 mg/kg	Improves focus, clarity, and memory	30–60 min before tasks
Anti-Aging and Longevity	1–2 mg/kg	Slows aging, reduces oxidative stress	Daily, with food
Recovery	1–2 mg/kg	Speeds physical and mental recovery	Post-stress or exercise
Therapeutic Applications	2–3 mg/kg	Supports brain health, combats chronic conditions	Under professional guidance

This quick-reference guide simplifies methylene blue's use, providing you with practical and actionable steps to meet your wellness goals. By understanding dosages, their effects, and when to use them, you can maximize the benefits of methylene blue safely and effectively. Pair this guide with consistent use and a healthy lifestyle to unlock its full potential.

RECOMMENDED PRODUCTS AND TRUSTED SOURCES

Selecting the right methylene blue product is crucial for safety, effectiveness, and achieving your wellness goals. With the growing interest in methylene blue, the market is filled with various options—but not all are created equal. This section guides you step-by-step on what to look for, trusted sources to consider, and tips to ensure you're choosing high-quality products.

Understanding Product Quality

The quality of methylene blue varies greatly depending on its intended use. Industrial-grade methylene blue, often used for dyeing or research, is not suitable for human consumption and can contain harmful impurities. Instead, look for *pharmaceutical or lab-grade methylene blue* that meets high safety and purity standards.

Key Features of a High-Quality Product:

1. **Purity:** Ensure the product has a purity of *99.9% or higher* to avoid contaminants.
2. **Third-Party Testing:** Look for products that are independently tested for heavy metals, additives, or impurities.
3. **Intended Use:** Confirm the product is labeled as safe for human consumption or cosmetic use, depending on your purpose.
4. **Transparency:** Reliable manufacturers provide clear information about ingredients, sourcing, and manufacturing processes.

Recommended Product Types

Depending on your goals and method of administration, there are different forms of methylene blue to consider.

1. **Oral or Sublingual Products**
    * **Best For:** General wellness, energy enhancement, cognitive support, and anti-aging.
    * **Features:** Available in liquid solutions or tablets specifically designed for human use.
    * **Example:** A pharmaceutical-grade methylene blue solution with no additives or stabilizers.

2. Topical Applications
    * **Best For:** Skin health, anti-aging, and localized treatment.
    * **Features:** Creams or serums containing methylene blue formulated for cosmetic use.
    * **Example:** Products combined with other skin-enhancing ingredients like hyaluronic acid or peptides.

3. **Innovative Delivery Systems**
   - **Best For:** Advanced users seeking targeted effects.
   - **Features:** Transdermal patches, time-release capsules, or nanoformulations for precision delivery.
   - **Example:** Patches offering controlled, steady absorption over several hours.

Trusted Sources

When purchasing methylene blue, choose suppliers known for quality and reliability. Below are some trusted categories of suppliers:

1. **Pharmaceutical Companies:** Companies specializing in lab-grade products often have stringent quality controls.
2. **Reputable Online Retailers:** Platforms with verified reviews and clear product descriptions. Look for customer testimonials and third-party certifications.
3. **Specialized Biohacking Stores:** Niche stores catering to the biohacking community often stock high-purity methylene blue and provide detailed usage instructions.

If I may offer a suggestion based on my personal experience with the product, here are the ASINs of the two best options available on Amazon. After trying several, I found these two to be the most reliable and effective.

What is an ASIN? An ASIN (Amazon Standard Identification Number) is a unique code assigned to every product on Amazon—think of it like a product's "social security number." Simply enter the ASIN code into Amazon's search bar, and it will take you directly to the product page.

- B09J1JRSLC
- B0BXTCGP6B

Safety Tips for Purchasing

1. **Avoid Industrial Products:** These are not safe for human use and can contain harmful additives.
2. **Read Reviews:** Check customer feedback to ensure consistency in product quality.
3. **Ask for Certificates of Analysis (COA):** Trusted suppliers will provide these documents to verify purity and safety.
4. **Start Small:** Purchase a small quantity first to test compatibility and effectiveness.

Decision-Making Table: Choosing the Best Methylene Blue Product

Criteria	What to Look For	Why It Matters	How to Evaluate
Purity	Minimum of 99.9% purity	Ensures the product is free from harmful contaminants or additives that could cause side effects.	Check the product label or ask for a Certificate of Analysis (COA) from the supplier.
Third-Party Testing	Verified independent lab tests confirming purity and safety	Verifies the product's claims and provides assurance of its quality.	Look for testing details on the supplier's website or product packaging.
Intended Use	Clearly labeled as safe for human consumption (or cosmetic use for topical applications)	Confirms the product's suitability for your intended application, such as oral, sublingual, or skin use.	Avoid products labeled industrial-grade or non-human use.
Manufacturer Reputation	Well-known, reputable manufacturers or suppliers with good customer feedback	Reputable manufacturers are more likely to adhere to strict quality and safety standards.	Research online reviews, check biohacking forums, or consult recommendations from health professionals.
Formulation	Matches your goals and preferred method of administration (e.g., solution, cream, capsule, patch)	Ensures the product aligns with your usage goals, such as energy enhancement, cognitive support, or skin health.	Compare options based on the delivery system best suited to your needs (e.g., liquid for oral use, cream for topical application).
Additives and Ingredients	Free from unnecessary stabilizers, preservatives, or heavy metals	Reduces the risk of side effects or interference with methylene blue's effectiveness.	Read the ingredient list carefully. Choose products with minimal additives or transparent formulations.
Customer Reviews	Positive reviews highlighting quality, effectiveness, and reliable results	Helps gauge real-world user experiences and satisfaction with the product.	Look for detailed customer reviews on retailer websites or biohacking communities.
Price	Fair pricing without compromising on quality	Avoids overspending while ensuring you're purchasing a high-quality product.	Compare prices per unit or dose across similar products. Be cautious of overly cheap products that may indicate lower quality.
Ease of Use	Convenient packaging and dosing instructions	Simplifies integration into your routine and prevents dosing errors.	Evaluate if the product includes a dropper, pre-measured capsules, or clear usage guidelines.
Return Policy	Flexible return or refund policy	Provides assurance in case the product doesn't meet expectations or has defects.	Check the supplier's return policy for clarity and ease of use.
Shipping and Availability	Fast, reliable shipping with consistent availability of stock	Ensures timely delivery and long-term access to the product if needed for ongoing use.	Look for clear shipping times and stock availability on the supplier's website or retailer platform.

How to Use This Table

1. **Identify Your Needs:** Clarify your goals (e.g., energy enhancement, skin health, or therapeutic use).
2. **Compare Products:** Use the criteria to evaluate multiple products of the same type.
3. **Score Each Product:** Assign a score (e.g., 1–5) to each criterion for each product, then total the scores to determine the best choice.
4. **Make an Informed Decision:** Select the product that best aligns with your goals, safety requirements, and budget.

This table provides a structured approach to help readers confidently choose the most suitable methylene blue product.

CONCLUSION: UNLOCKING THE POWER OF METHYLENE BLUE

As we reach the end of this journey, the transformative potential of methylene blue becomes clear. More than a supplement, methylene blue is a tool—a gateway to lifelong wellness and a healthier, more empowered life. Its unique ability to enhance cellular energy, support brain health, combat aging, and address chronic conditions places it at the forefront of modern health optimization. Let's take a moment to reflect on the key takeaways from this book and how they can inspire you to take action.

EMBRACING METHYLENE BLUE AS A TOOL FOR LIFELONG WELLNESS

Throughout this book, we've explored the incredible potential of methylene blue to revolutionize health and wellness. From enhancing energy and cognition to supporting longevity and recovery, methylene blue stands as a unique tool to address the core challenges of aging and modern health. But more than just a supplement, methylene blue represents an opportunity to take control of your well-being and unlock your full potential.

1. **A Recap of Key Benefits:** Methylene blue's versatility lies in its ability to target the root causes of many health challenges:
   - **Boosts Cellular Energy:** By enhancing mitochondrial efficiency, methylene blue increases ATP production, giving you sustained energy to power through your day.
   - **Sharpens Mental Clarity:** Supporting brain health, it improves focus, memory, and overall cognitive performance, helping you stay sharp at any age.
   - **Slows Aging:** By reducing oxidative stress and supporting cellular repair, methylene blue combats the effects of aging at a cellular level.
   - **Supports Recovery:** Its anti-inflammatory and energy-enhancing properties accelerate recovery from physical and mental stress.
   - **Addresses Chronic Conditions:** From neurodegenerative diseases to immune health, methylene blue's potential extends to some of the most complex health challenges we face today.

These benefits are not isolated—they form a foundation for lifelong wellness. By integrating methylene blue into your routine, you are proactively working to maintain vitality, resilience, and balance.

2. **A Tool for Empowerment:** Methylene blue is not just about addressing symptoms; it's about empowerment. It provides a way to take control of your health, offering measurable improvements that build confidence in your ability to shape your well-being. Unlike conventional treatments that often focus on short-term fixes, methylene blue works at the root level, supporting the body's natural processes and resilience. Incorporating methylene blue into your life is also an opportunity to embrace the broader philosophy of biohacking. By understanding how your body works and using science-backed tools to optimize it, you can achieve a level of health and performance that might have once seemed out of reach.

3. **Making It a Lifelong Habit:** Building a wellness routine that includes methylene blue is straightforward:
    - **Start with a Clear Goal:** Whether it's more energy, sharper focus, or better aging, define what you want to achieve.
    - **Begin Small:** Use the dosage guidelines from this book to start safely, tracking how your body responds.
    - **Combine with Healthy Practices:** Pair methylene blue with complementary habits like a nutrient-rich diet, regular exercise, and mindfulness practices for amplified effects.
    - **Stay Consistent:** Lifelong wellness comes from daily habits. Make methylene blue a part of your routine and give it time to work.

4. **A Call to Action:** Your journey doesn't end here—it begins. Methylene blue is your ally in the quest for lifelong wellness, but it's up to you to take the first step. Begin experimenting, track your progress, and embrace the process of optimizing your health. You hold the power to shape your future. By embracing methylene blue and the philosophy of biohacking, you're not just adding years to your life—you're adding life to your years. Start today, and unlock the healthier, more vibrant version of yourself that's waiting.

ENCOURAGEMENT FOR CONTINUED EXPLORATION AND OPTIMIZATION

As we close this chapter of your journey with methylene blue, it's important to recognize that this is just the beginning. The true power of methylene blue lies not only in its proven benefits but also in its ability to inspire continuous learning, experimentation, and growth. Your journey toward optimal health and wellness is a dynamic process, and methylene blue is a tool that evolves with you.

Reflecting on What You've Learned

Throughout this book, you've gained a comprehensive understanding of methylene blue's potential to transform your health:
- It boosts energy by improving mitochondrial function, helping you power through life with vitality.

- It sharpens mental clarity and focus, enhancing productivity and cognitive resilience.
- It supports longevity by addressing cellular aging, reducing oxidative stress, and promoting repair.
- It aids recovery from stress and physical exertion, ensuring you're ready for whatever challenges come your way.
- It offers therapeutic potential for chronic conditions, from neurodegenerative diseases to immune health.

These benefits form a foundation for a healthier, more empowered life. Yet, the key to unlocking their full potential lies in your willingness to keep exploring and optimizing.

The Mindset of Exploration

Health optimization isn't a one-size-fits-all approach. It's about finding what works for you, understanding your unique body, and adapting your practices over time. Methylene blue is more than just a supplement—it's a gateway to a mindset of curiosity and self-discovery. By experimenting safely and tracking your progress, you'll uncover insights that can guide you toward even greater levels of wellness.

- **Be Open to Innovation:** Science continues to uncover new uses for methylene blue, from advanced delivery systems to groundbreaking therapeutic applications. Stay curious and embrace emerging research as it becomes available.
- **Experiment Wisely:** Begin with small, controlled changes in dosage or application methods, and observe how your body responds. This iterative process ensures that your approach remains both effective and safe.

Integrating Biohacking Principles

Methylene blue is a core tool in the broader philosophy of biohacking—a lifestyle dedicated to optimizing mind and body through science and self-awareness. By integrating methylene blue into a larger framework of biohacking practices, you can achieve synergistic benefits.

- **Combine with Other Biohacks:** Explore complementary strategies like red light therapy, NAD+ supplementation, intermittent fasting, or mindfulness techniques to amplify methylene blue's effects.
- **Leverage Technology:** Use wearable devices, apps, or journals to track metrics such as energy levels, sleep quality, or cognitive performance, helping you fine-tune your approach.
- **Adopt a Growth Mindset:** View your wellness journey as an ongoing process of discovery, where each step brings you closer to your full potential.

A Call to Action

The path to lifelong health and wellness is paved with curiosity and action. Methylene blue offers a proven starting point, but the real transformation happens when you take ownership of your journey.

<u>Begin today:</u>

- Experiment with methylene blue using the guidance provided in this book.
- Stay informed about new developments and research.
- Share your experiences to inspire and learn from others in the wellness community.

This is your moment to take charge of your health, embrace the philosophy of biohacking, and unlock your full potential. The journey is yours to define, and methylene blue is here to support you every step of the way. Now is the time to begin.

Your journey with methylene blue is an invitation to unlock your full potential. It's a chance to not only improve your health but to redefine what wellness means for you. With methylene blue as a cornerstone of your routine and a commitment to lifelong learning, you have the tools to achieve resilience, vitality, and balance. Take the first step. Experiment, explore, and embrace the possibilities. Your best self is waiting, and methylene blue can help you get there. The journey to lifelong wellness starts now—step boldly into your future.

GET YOUR GIFTS

It's time to unlock the exclusive bonuses promised on the cover! Gain access to extra content, unique recipes, and—most importantly—every tip, trick, and secret I've uncovered through years of mastering this incredible product.

The best part? It's just a quick scan away. Use your smartphone to scan the QR code and claim your exclusive bonuses instantly.

You deserve to feel your best and live well, take charge of your health today!

NOW IT'S YOUR TURN!

As we reach the end of this book, our journey together is far from over. Now it's your turn to make a meaningful impact. With just a few seconds of your time, you can make a big difference by leaving a simple review on Amazon.

Your feedback not only supports my work but also helps me improve the quality of my books and create even better content in the future. Your support isn't just valuable—it's truly essential.

Leaving a review is quick and easy. Simply grab your phone, scan the QR code, and share your thoughts about the book.

Thank you from the bottom of my heart for being a part of this journey. Your support means the world to me.

With gratitude,
Elvira

Made in the USA
Middletown, DE
27 April 2025

74815563R00044